PRAISE FOR PREVIOUS EDITIONS OF
ANSWERING YOUR QUESTIONS ABOUT HEART DISEASE AND SEX

Editor's Choice, iUniverse

Finalist in *ForeWord* Magazine's 2004 Book of the Year Awards

"A sensitive topic, ever so elegantly handled."
> — Judith Coche, Ph.D.
> Founder and Director of The Coche Center

"A book written with humoristic and didactic brilliance."
> — Frank Perez-Rivas, M.D., M.B.A.
> Retired Director of Oakland Park Veterans Administration Clinic

"I have not seen a more inspiring and integrative work on the connections between health, intimacy, and happiness. This book is a true celebration of the enduring human heart and spirit!"
> — Scott E. Borrelli, Ed.D.
> Director of Counseling Services, The American Intercontinental University of London
> Professor, University of Maryland
> Chief Editor, *The EMDR Practitioner*

"Dr. Chapunoff's superb book is a godsend for the 59 million Americans who have cardiovascular disease. With its easy to understand writing style, its poignant clinical vignettes, and its solid medical advice, this

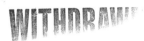

book deserves to be widely read and recommended."
— Aline Zoldbrod, Ph.D., Sex Therapist
Author of *Sex Smart*, a *ForeWord* Magazine Award Winner

"…There are no other books addressing the issues he covers. Dr. Chapunoff has opened the door to a long-neglected subject. He is honest and forthright with his answers. This excellent resource proves that an informative and educational reading experience can also be engaging even when the subject matter is very serious."
— Betty Corbin Tucker
Author of *The Thorn of Sexual Abuse*

"…Dr. Chapunoff examines the questions of heart disease and sex from every angle, both medical and personal. The information is timely, thoroughly researched, and highly relevant. The author provides a knowledgeable and caring approach to an important topic. Highly recommended!"
— Raymond C. Rosen, Ph.D.
Professor of Psychiatry and Medicine, R. W. Johnson Medical School
Director of Human Sexuality Program

"This book is a fun, interesting read, employing a lot of humor and great anecdotes. And it's got to be a more relevant read for the cardiac patient than the week-old *Better Homes & Gardens* in the hospital room. Forget the $20 get-well bouquet; give your convalescent a sex life for $15.95."
— John Huetter
Critic, *Boca Raton News*

"…Filled with amusing anecdotes and intricate explanations, this book is of value to anyone who has a sex drive and a beating heart."

> — Jacqueline Sousa
> Editor, *Coral Gables Living*

"This book takes the mystique out of heart disease and has the potential for becoming a well-thumbed reference book."

> — Karl Kunkel
> Critic, *ForeWord Magazine*

"Dr. Chapunoff offers the balm of simple clarity, compassion, and rock-solid guidance. There's a reason Dr. Chapunoff is held in such high regard…his skill, his writing, and his guidance are totally approachable, gentle, and wise."

> — Bernie Ahearn
> Radio Host of "A Man's World," Detroit, Michigan

© 2007 Eduardo Chapunoff

www.dreduardochapunoff.com

Library of Congress Cataloging-in-Publication Data

Chapunoff, Eduardo, 1936-
  Answering your questions about heart disease and sex / Eduardo Chapunoff ; foreword by Arnold A. Lazarus.
    p. cm.
  Includes index.
  ISBN-13: 978-1-57826-255-7
  1. Coronary heart disease--Complications. 2. Coronary heart disease--Patients--Sexual activity. 3. Heart--Diseases--Complications. 4. Heart--Diseases--Patients--Sexual acitivity. I. Title.
  RC685.C6C4537 2007
  616.1'23--dc22
                          2007022620

Cover design by Farrimond New York
Interior design by Jacinta Monniere, Jasmine Cordoza, and Allison Furrer
Published in the United States
10 9 8 7 6 5 4 3 2 1

ANSWERING
YOUR QUESTIONS ABOUT
HEART DISEASE AND
SEX

EDUARDO CHAPUNOFF, M.D., F.A.C.P., F.A.C.C.

FOREWORD BY
ARNOLD A. LAZARUS, PH.D.
DISTINGUISHED PROFESSOR EMERITUS
OF PSYCHOLOGY, RUTGERS UNIVERSITY

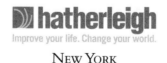

Improve your life. Change your world.

NEW YORK

419660

Dedication

In loving memory of my parents,
Julio and Jacinta,
and to my wife and angel,
Cristina

Contents

Foreword

There is much to be learned by reading this book. Dr. Chapunoff's work is a cleverly intertwined exposition on sexuality and heart disease. The nuances and complexities of the doctor–patient relationship are skillfully presented in a user-friendly manner, and there are many hilarious dialogues that shed light on "human nature" and show what doctors and patients have to contend with.

Who can benefit from this book? Almost everyone! Any literate individual with an interest in his or her health, and specifically anyone who wants to know more about love, life, hearts, sex, compassion, and human relationships, will find this book of enormous value. Professionals can also derive benefit from Dr. Chapunoff's vast experience and profound wisdom. I would like to see *Answering Your Questions About Heart Disease and Sex* on recommended reading lists in medical schools, clinical psychology departments, and in all facilities that train people to be health providers.

Many people incorrectly believe that most doctors have a broad state-of-the-art knowledge on matters pertaining to exercise, nutrition, sex, personal relationships, and psychology. In fact, physicians learn a good deal about anatomy, physiology, and biochemistry, and their medical curriculum focuses primarily on the diagnosis, treatment, and management of various physical illnesses. It is only recently that formal training in such topics as the doctor–patient relationship, nutrition, and health maintenance have been part of a physician's training, and the extent and quality of these topics varies from school to school.

A few years ago, a 34-year-old obstetrician–gynecologist consulted me for two main problems: 1) He was about to get married and felt ambivalent about this decision. 2) When patients asked him about sexual matters, he felt awkward and blushed so visibly that several women apologized for having embarrassed him.

He claimed to be quite comfortable engaging in sexual relations with his fiancée (and several other women before her), and he experienced no discomfiture when examining his patients. But when a patient, two months after suffering a heart attack, asked him if it would be safe for her to resume having sexual intercourse, and whether it would be harmful for her to masturbate, he blushed and told her to discuss this with her cardiologist. The woman said she already had done so, but the cardiologist had offhandedly said that she should know what she felt capable of doing. What a far cry from the wit, good judgment, empathy, humor, and knowledge that Dr. Chapunoff displays. As soon as this book is published, I will make sure to send a copy to my former OBGYN patient, his patient who had the heart attack, and her cardiologist.

The word that comes immediately to mind about *Answering Your Questions About Heart Disease and Sex* is "affirmative." It empowers one with a well-seasoned map of how to enhance and take charge of important aspects of medical and psychological health and well-being. It makes me wish with all my heart that Dr. Chapunoff was my personal physician.

— Arnold A. Lazarus, Ph.D., A.B.P.P.
Distinguished Professor Emeritus of Psychology, Rutgers University

Introduction

Sex, the Heart, and the Search for Happiness

Two people starting a conversation:

"Let me introduce you to the subject of sex."

"The pleasure is mine!"

This book is an extended version of *Sex and the Cardiac Patient: A Practical Guide,* which I published in English and Spanish in 1991. It sold in the United States and other countries, some as distant as Singapore and Australia. I held radio and TV interviews, and distinguished professionals and journalists offered favorable comments. People whom I had never met but had read the book, consulted me by mail and telephone. The experience was both very interesting and spiritually rewarding. I learned that patients with sexual concerns can present their problems to a professional who inspires confidence—even if they don't know him or her personally. In fact, when the consulting doctor's face is not seen, some patients suffering from sexual dysfunctions are less inhibited and may describe intimate conflicts in more detail and more accurately. I had this experience with phone calls and letters I received from patients I never met.

Complaints about patient–physician communication seem to be the same today as they were a decade ago: "The doctor doesn't have enough time;" "He/she is too busy;" "I'd like to open up and talk, but I don't know how or where to start;" "I'm not asked any questions."

SHYNESS AND INHIBITIONS

Embarrassment has always been a problem. I'll never forget the contrasting views of two female patients. One told me: "I feel terrible talking to my doctor about sex. I've known him for such a short time." The other woman said: "I can't imagine myself discussing sexual details with my doctor. I've known him for such a long time. He's like a relative. I don't like to talk about intimacies with members of my family."

For most people, talking about sex with a doctor is as difficult today as it was 100 years ago—and it's likely to remain that way.

Shortly following the publication of my previous book, I received a number of phone calls from cardiac patients who had sexual concerns, but their shyness overwhelmed them. The wife of an elderly gentleman called my office, and we had this exchange:

"Hello, may I help you?"

"Are you Dr. Chapunoff?"

"Yes, Madam, I am."

"I understand you wrote a book called Sex and the Cardiac Patient. Is that true?"

"Yes, Madam, it is."

"My husband is a senior citizen, 83, and to be perfectly honest, I'm no spring chicken either. Do you understand that?"

"Yes, I do."

"We are having problems. Do you get that?"

"I'm trying, Madam. What kind of problems, may I ask?"

"Problems, problems."

"Oh, I see. I'll be happy to give you an appointment."

"An appointment? Who wants an appointment? We don't want an appointment. We don't want an examination, either. My husband would never agree to see a doctor for this. And I'm just about the same. It's awful. We don't know how to talk about these things."

"If that's the case, would you like to ask me a question? Perhaps I could give you some guidance."

"Yes, I'd like to ask you a very simple question."

"In that case, I'm warning you: I might come up with a very simple answer."

"That's okay. I understand. This is the question: My husband and I are both cardiac patients. We want to know if we can sleep together."

"Well, let me tell you this: I think you can sleep together, but I don't know if you should."

Conversations about sex between patients and doctors (except for psychiatrists and psychologists) are frequently evasive. A combination of discomfort and bias frequently separates them. Recovering cardiac patients are curious to know when they can make love, which positions are preferable, and whether they should be admonished or congratulated for masturbating. After a heart attack or any other cardiac crisis, they wait in vain for the doctor's blessing to resume sexual activity. If there is no blessing, they still look for guidance, and watch for a hopeful signal, maybe even a wink, anything that resembles a sign of approval to go back to the good old days. Finally, nature takes its course. Couples stumble back into some kind of sexual pattern, but without the needed counseling and reassurances.

AN UNEXPECTED INVITATION

Some years ago, while I was working at my office, I received a call from a Miami TV station requesting my participation in a program entitled "Sex and Cardiovascular Health." At the time, I had too many commitments, so I proposed that they postpone the program for a couple of months. I didn't know why I'd been selected since I'd never written or lectured on the subject. In any event, the station didn't call me back, and the interview never took place. (I'm still grateful for that.)

An interesting aftermath of this incident was my reaction to it. After the initial excitement mellowed, I began to wonder how much I really knew about sex and cardiovascular diseases. I prepared a test with a number of questions. I took it, and guess what? I flunked it with honors. These were some of the questions I had raised: "Do I really know how to advise cardiac patients about precautions they should take before, during, and after sexual intercourse?" "Following a massive heart attack, when should a person be able to resume sexual activity, and then, what special positions, if any, he or she should be recommended to use?" "How dangerous is it for patients with hypertension, heart failure, valvular heart disease, aortic aneurysm and/or cardiac rhythm disturbances to engage in passionate lovemaking? Would the risk be low or prohibitive?" And so forth. It was immediately obvious to me that I had never paid special attention to the subject, and I had homework to do.

I began the search for information on sex and the cardiac patient in classical medical and cardiology textbooks; I didn't find any information.

Articles in medical journals were few and far between.

An enormous volume has been written about cardiac disorders, and publications about sex are almost as abundant as the number of living spermatozoa. Yet, two basic issues were infrequently addressed: one, the effects of sex on cardiac patients, and two, the consequences of heart disease on sexual functioning.

Fortunately, in the past decade there have been important publications in medical journals addressing those issues. Until recently, however, scientifically speaking, this field was in a near-virginal state.

New knowledge has been gained by doing clinical research and clinical observations of patients with heart disease and their sexual performance. To begin with, new medicines and treatment modalities dealing with angina, congestive heart failure, hypertension, evaluation and treatment of disabling or life-threatening arrhythmias by ablation and intracardiac defibrillators, improved prosthetic heart valves, methods to prevent and treat acute and chronic cardiac conditions have become available and are widely used.

Many coronary bypass surgeries are currently being avoided and have been replaced by balloon angioplasty (dilatation of a narrowed artery) and implantation of stents to keep those arteries open. This has effectively shortened the length of hospitalization and reduced patients' discomforts and accelerated the recovery process. A coronary angioplasty usually takes one day in the hospital, with minor discomfort. Cardiac surgery demands a few days in the hospital and longer recuperation time.

All of the above have changed for the better the dynamics of the cardiac patient's sexual interaction.

Psychotherapists have also reviewed and replaced old psychoanalytic techniques with innovative, modern schools of thought that provide psychological counseling and drug therapy faster and more effectively.

Urologists have improved penile prosthesis for a selective patient population, and women with sexual dysfunctions involving desire, arousal, orgasmic, or sexual pain disorders are being more specifically treated by gynecologists with expertise in this area.

The introduction of Viagra in 1998, followed by Levitra and Cialis, has made a dramatic difference in male and female intimate experiences. Although not all who take these medications respond with an erection and/or adequate tolerance, unquestionably, they are very helpful.

Answering Your Questions about Heart Disease and Sex discusses multiple concerns that directly or indirectly relate to cardiac patients and their sexual partners. It is difficult to tell you which are more important. To me, all of them are. Things that you've never focused on and perhaps considered trivial, may, in reality, be decisive for your cardiac health and sexuality. At times, just a single but important risk factor, poorly managed, may cause heart disease, impotence, and loss of life. Smoking is a typical example. Information that is very important for the preservation of your cardiovascular health and sexual functioning has been included in the Appendix section at the back of the book. Please keep in mind that this is an educational guide and not a substitute for any of your doctor's recommendations. Medical treatments are provided by doctors, not books. What you learn here, however, may help you initiate or expand the dialogue with your physician and your domestic partner.

Throughout the book, there are anecdotal experiences that illustrate that the sex life of cardiac patients is neither as complicated as some imagine, nor as simple as others would like it to be.

While this work focuses on heterosexual sex, the same advice and cautions apply equally to gay men and lesbians with heart disease.

Any book on sex is controversial. I anticipate that for some people my book will fall into this category, too. That's unavoidable. There are probably no two people in the entire world who think and feel alike about sexuality. Each individual's sexuality is like his or her fingerprints or DNA: unique.

Some of my views may seem unconventional. I have a tendency to be direct and straightforward, and you'll probably notice this as you read some of my comments and read the way I conduct interviews with my patients. The material is sprinkled with humor. (I'm not sure humor can make you live longer, but it can certainly make you live better).

HOW MANY PEOPLE ARE INVOLVED?

There are 59 million Americans who suffer from cardiovascular diseases. The two most frequent diseases are hypertension (high blood pressure) and heart disease. Atherosclerosis (thickening or hardening of the arteries that result in blockages) is the basis for most cardiovascular diseases, and it involves the coronary arteries (coronary artery disease), the carotid-cerebral circulation (strokes), and multiple arterial territories, such as the arteries of the gut, those supplying blood to the kidneys, genitals, and lower extremities.

The thoracic and abdominal aorta may have portions that become enlarged, usually due to a combination of hypertension and atherosclerosis. These are called "aneurysms."

In the past three decades there has been a gradual decrease in cardiovascular mortality, but these diseases continue to be the most common cause of death and disability, accounting for one in five deaths annually.

Coronary heart disease is the leading cause of death in both men and women and in every racial and ethnic group, except in Asian-American women, where it is cancer.

In the United States, there are approximately 1.1 million heart attacks (myocardial infarctions) each year. About 650,000 are new, and 450,000 are recurrent heart attacks. A full 33 percent of all heart attacks go unrecognized. That means a heart attack occurs but evades recognition (by patient, doctor, or both). Half of the unrecognized myocardial infarctions show no symptoms. These are called "silent" heart attacks.

The death rate is 50 percent higher in blacks than in whites in the age group 35 to 44—a difference that narrows with increasing age and disappears by age 75. Coronary mortality is not as high in Hispanics as it is among blacks and whites.

The percentage of sudden coronary deaths that occur without previously diagnosed coronary artery disease is much greater in women than in men.

Hypertension affects 58 million Americans, and about 15 million of them are not even aware they have it. Annually, hypertension contributes to 600,000 strokes, nearly one million heart attacks, and 400,000 new cases of congestive heart failure. Hundreds of thousands also suffer from hypertension-induced kidney failure.

About 4.8 million Americans have heart failure (weakening of the heart muscle). Add in the cases of valvular heart disease, cardiomyopathies (chronic diseases of the heart muscle), cardiac rhythm abnormalities (called arrhythmias or dysrrhythmias), rheumatic heart disease, congenital lesions, pulmonary thromboembolism (clots that form in the lower extremities that travel to the lungs), and the end result is millions who suffer and become disabled, and hundreds of thousands who lose their lives. And we are just referring to the United States. What about the rest of the world? The numbers are staggering.

WHAT CAN YOU DO?

First, become familiar with the nature and extent of your cardiac and general medical conditions. Should sexual function be affected, it's important to assess that too. The cooperation of your sexual partner is essential.

Learn basic concepts about the circulatory system in health and disease, and about sexuality, nutrition, stress control, treatment options, and so on. The prevalence and mortality from cardiovascular disease increases with decreasing levels of education. A little knowledge could prolong your life. Greater knowledge might save it.

Nowadays, medicine is practiced differently than it was just a few decades ago. The old practitioner used to spend more time talking to patients and holding their hands, providing spiritual comfort. Remember those memorable house calls? A family doctor was the clinician, the psychologist, the psychiatrist, the obstetrician, the pediatrician, and sometimes, even the surgeon. Those days are gone. The winds of modern times blew them away. But don't feel too badly. The good news is that when you have a heart attack, you're quickly monitored at the Emergency Room or Intensive Care Unit, and although the physician doesn't always hold your hand, he or she gives you a clot-dissolving medication or opens up a clogged coronary artery, saving your life in the process.

As far as the communication issue goes, if you have problems in this area address them as soon as you can. Start by trying to achieve successful communication with yourself. Become your own best friend to learn who you really are. You may think you know. You may be right, you may be wrong. This requires introspection, a little time to think or meditate, perhaps a few productive sessions with a good psychotherapist. Analyze your surroundings (spouse, family, work environment, financial status). Look for specific solutions.

Don't feel uncomfortable when talking about sex, do it in a natural way, and try to overcome any barriers that limit conversations with your physician. Think positively. There are excellent reasons to be optimistic:

Science has never before offered so many treatment alternatives and technological advances.

Understandably, a measure of realism and acceptance of some bumps along the road to recovery are needed. A return to sexual engagement should not be rushed, but stagnation is also to be avoided. Undue delays are known to trigger nervous tension, anxiety, and on occasion, some ugliness of disposition as well.

As we can see, cardiovascular disease and sexual dysfunctions have enough power to adversely affect personal and family relations, work performance, productivity, mental health, and leisure-time pursuits. Before you continue the journey through the pages of this book, remember: if problems exist, so do solutions. Try to find them. Lovemaking, after all, is too important to be ignored. And for those who suffer socio-economic hardships in many areas of the world, and don't have available resources to improve their lives, we can only hope that one day, they will materialize their dreams, and that will include, of course, the happiness of their intimate experiences. Good sex is something that people like thinking about, when other elementary needs (food, housing, and their children's well-being) are secured. When extreme poverty and deprivation prevail, good sex, careful sex, romantic sex, lusty sex, and even lousy sex, become a luxury. Shouldn't we all dream of the day when everybody, poor and affluent, will be able to learn to take care of themselves, avoid heart attacks and strokes, and have terrific sex? And then, after enjoying a night of glorious intimacy, they'd take to the streets— smiling, jumping, dancing, and singing in the rain, Gene Kelly-style— screaming to everybody who passes by, in the happiest possible way, "What a beautiful day this is!"

PART ONE

AN INTRODUCTION TO SEX AND THE HEART

Chapter 1

A New Beginning: The Good Side of Your Crisis

HUSBAND: "Darling, the heart attack has transformed me into a totally different person. Do you agree?"

WIFE: "Yes, I do...and I think it's wonderful!"

Let's face it: Heart attacks, or impending ones that were prevented or minimized by opportune medical intervention, are traumatic experiences. So are other heart conditions, such as cardiomyopathies (weak heart muscle), diseases of the heart valves, life-threatening arrhythmias, significant accumulation of fluid in the pericardium, clots traveling from the leg veins to the lungs (pulmonary emboli), and congenital heart disease, among many others.

Following recovery from an unexpected cardiac event, you are not the same person. Becoming a different individual, however, is not always as bad as it sounds. Sometimes it is desirable, and occasionally, it is lifesaving. The crucial point, then, is not being different, but being better.

Unquestionably, adversity teaches us more than pleasure does. We learn more during minutes or hours of suffering than during years of joy. If you learn to adjust, limit your anguish and sensitivity, and develop the ability to practice damage control following setbacks, you'll look at life from a different perspective. You'll be stronger and more determined than ever to be happy and at peace with yourself and the rest of the world.

A cardiac crisis claims a price: physically, emotionally, and financially. Repercussive waves spread throughout your psyche, your spouse's and your children's psyches, your credit cards, and what used to be your savings account. At home, a worrisome uncertainty permeates the air.

If you had cardiac surgery, you came out of the operating room with so many strange devices—thoracic tubes draining blood, an endotracheal tube, intravenous and intra-arterial lines, bladder catheter, bandages all over—that rather than a patient, you looked more like an astronaut ready for a mission to another planet.

A few days later, you began to ask yourself how long it would take to recover your health and physical stamina, your financial base, and your sexual functioning. You realized that a new philosophy and radical lifestyle changes had become essential priorities.

For years—most of your life, actually—you've consumed the wrong food, carried too much weight, and had abnormal blood levels of cholesterol. Your blood pressure was checked every blue moon, and your regular exercise consisted of moving two fingers on the computer board at least eight hours a day. Smoking didn't help much either. And then there was the struggle of long-standing, unresolved personal and family conflicts.

A drastic change demands mental reprogramming. Unless you do that and develop a well-structured, carefully planned strategy that you implement with self-discipline in a consistent way, you'll repeat the same mistakes, perpetuate the same behavioral patterns, and jeopardize the health and safety of your cardiovascular system.

Not every unpleasant encounter with destiny impacts us negatively. Wisely managed, even ugly situations can be an eventual source of happiness. You need willpower, assertiveness, and determination. If you feel you are missing those qualities, that's okay too; you can still develop them.

Benefits from getting sick? Is this a joke? Not at all. A very ignorant man was once asked if he believed in ghosts, and he answered: "I certainly don't believe in ghosts, although I'm positive they do exist!"

After reading the next few pages, I hope you'll reach the same conclusion.

BENEFIT ONE
A Cardiac Crisis = New Knowledge = A Safer Future
1. Your cardiac crisis taught you more in a few days than you learned in decades prior.
2. The results of diagnostic tests have let you know the extent of your disease and how to deal with it.
3. That knowledge will enable you and your doctor to treat your condition effectively.

The combination of 1, 2, and 3 equals safety.

If you survived a heart attack or cardiac surgery (and obviously you did, otherwise you wouldn't be reading this book), you are far more protected than legions of individuals who believe that they are healthy and who don't know that they have a critical obstruction of a coronary artery. They are attending parties, cheerfully celebrating their successful businesses or careers, playing tennis, and don't suspect that in the next days or weeks, they'll have a heart attack, or worse. Each year, 250,000 people die suddenly of acute heart attacks in the United States. These people don't reach the hospital alive.

Your newly acquired knowledge is the best insurance you can get against such an outcome.

BENEFIT TWO
Sometimes, Having A Heart Attack Is Better Than Not Having One

Is there anything wrong with this statement? What does it mean? Can having a heart attack be preferable to not having one? The answer is a resounding YES!

Let me clarify this: An acute myocardial infarction results from the sudden blockage of a coronary artery by a blood clot. The blood supply to the heart muscle is cut off, and the muscle gets damaged. This process takes anywhere from twenty minutes to hours. At times, however, and in just a few seconds, an acutely blocked coronary artery causes ventricular fibrillation (rapid, irregular, and extremely weak contractions of the muscle fibers of the heart). This chaotic rhythm produces no effective cardiac contractions. As a result, no blood is ejected from the heart. Unless cardiac resuscitation restores an adequate rhythm and cardiac pumping function, the outcome is fatal. The development of ventricular fibrillation can occur so quickly that the heart does not have enough time to develop an acute myocardial infarction (heart attack). Instead, the person is killed by an electrical disturbance, much like the one produced by lightening.

Now, given a choice, wouldn't you rather have an acute myocardial infarction and survive it (after all, most patients do), than have no myocardial infarction, but a sudden death induced by a nasty rhythm called ventricular fibrillation? Of course, you would.

BENEFIT THREE
Prevention of Strokes, Heart Failure, and Kidney Damage

Thanks to your heart attack and the educational process that resulted from it, you've learned that having low blood pressure is much better than having high blood pressure (hypertension). High blood pressure leads to strokes, heart failure, and kidney damage. You've probably heard that before, but never paid too much attention to the concept. Years ago, your blood pressure was elevated, you took medications for a while, and seldom checked your pressure afterwards.

Now you have committed yourself to having your blood pressure checked regularly, and you are aware that abnormal elevations are not acceptable.

BENEFIT FOUR
Prevention of Emphysema, Chronic Bronchitis, and Lung, Throat, Tongue, Esophageal, and Pancreatic Cancer

Smoking is a lethal sport. If your heart attack motivated you to give up this vice, be thankful. You may avoid disability or death from lung disease or any of the cancers mentioned above.

Your heart attack was a flashing red light, warning you about the dangers yet to come from smoking. It prevented you from getting into future, deeper trouble.

Quite often, the damage caused by smoking in the lungs, the heart, and other organs, such as the various cancers I mentioned above, is directly proportional to the length and amount of smoking. A person who quits the habit because he or she had an acute myocardial infarction at age 50, may well avoid emphysema, shortness of breath, chronic cough, and cancer at age 60.

BENEFIT FIVE
Prevention of Erectile Failure
Atherosclerosis affects many arteries, not just coronary arteries. By correcting the various risk factors that lead to hardening of the arteries, you're doing your best to avoid plaques that can block the pelvic arteries (lower abdomen). That will contribute to the prevention of sexual dysfunctions in females and males.

BENEFIT SIX
Dividends of Losing Weight
Your recent heart crisis motivated you to change eating habits and avoid a sedentary lifestyle. Normalization of your weight will reduce the severity of heart disease and diabetes, help regulate cholesterol levels, protect against degenerative changes in the lower back, knees, and ankle joints, and prevent blood clots in the veins of the legs, which can travel to the lungs and have serious consequences, such as pulmonary emboli.

BENEFIT SEVEN
Working Fewer Hours More Productively
Years ago, I had a 50-year-old patient, Joe, who owned a restaurant. He worked 16 hours a day and was as busy as a beaver. Holidays and weekends didn't exist for him. He suffered from high blood pressure but never found the time to check it—or treat it. He stopped working the day he landed in the emergency room.

Joe recovered from his coronary attack but couldn't work for about 3 months. He was unable to supervise his business and lost his income. During an office visit, he described to me his desperate situation. In one of my desk drawers, I had kept a book on real estate techniques—

specifically, on how to invest with limited resources. On a whim, I gave it to him.

It seemed the book was written for Joe. In a short time, he tripled his income, yet he worked much less. He kept on thanking his heart attack for changing his life.

While I certainly do not specialize in financial counseling, this time my advice proved to be more effective than some of my medical treatments.

BENEFIT EIGHT
More Leisure Time

The old hurried schedule is gone. Good for you! You have finally decided to listen to your favorite music and read those books you always wanted to read but never had time for. You are also taking weekends off, planning regular vacations, and playing golf. When was the last time you had it so good?

BENEFIT NINE
A Better Family Life

Slowing down will allow you more time with your family. You'll find refuge in special moments with your spouse and children. Before your coronary event, you worked so long and so hard that you had little time to share with your loved ones. Your kids barely saw you, and there were communication failures. Now, you'll all be eating at the dinner table again, you'll talk to your children about their schoolwork, and you'll play with them. You'll get to know each other—and that's the way it should be.

BENEFIT TEN
Renewed Appreciation of Life

Surviving your cardiac illness brought you a new awareness. In a way, you're rediscovering the meaning of life. Every day is precious, every moment counts. You are enjoying the sunshine, the taste of grapes, the meaning of love, the charm of a puppy, and the geniality of Mozart. You've reached a new dimension, and with it, the beginning of a new sensation: the sensation of being alive.

As you can see, you can profit from having a cardiac crisis. That does not mean that I recommend everyone have a coronary attack just to enjoy the listed benefits. But if you went through such an ordeal, I suggest you look not only at the losses it caused, but the renewed opportunities. By learning to cope with adversity and amend past errors, you'll come to realize that the benefits I described are real, and not a bunch of aimless abstractions thrown into the wind.

Chapter 2

Cardiovascular Disease, Sex, and Aging

SENIOR CITIZEN TO A FRIEND: "Joe, with respect to sex: Do you buy the idea that sexual potency and sexual experience are equally important?"

JOE: "Oh yeah, I sure do. Just give me a pound of each!"

Wines get better with age, or so they say. With advancing age, we do too—within limits, of course. As time goes by, things change: the skin shows some wrinkles, joints become stiffer, muscles aren't so strong, the hair gets brittle (when there's some left), and at some point, the genitals begin to believe in miracles. But, wait a minute! Let's be careful about generalizations, characterizations, and misleading stereotypes. Not only do many seniors perform very well—mentally, physically, and sexually—but they also perform far better than individuals 30 years younger.

Unquestionably, aging does not affect everybody the same way. Each individual possesses his or her own genetic code and unique set of environmental influences. These two factors matter a great deal.

If you are lucky—and I mean plain lucky—and you were born with superior genes that transmit longevity and natural immunity to a number of vascular, infectious, tumoral, and other ailments, you have a very good chance of living a long and healthy life. That is, of course, if you haven't messed up your body tissues and chemistry with smoking, booze, chronic aggravation, French fries, and other undesirable items.

The important thing, however, is not to delve into the past—about which you can do nothing—but to figure out where you stand health-wise, right now. The focus here is on cardiovascular assessment and its possible implications for your sexuality.

THE CARDIOVASCULAR MACHINE

PATIENT: "Doc, do you believe in trying not to fix something that ain't broken?"

PHYSICIAN: "Yes, I do...but I also believe in preventing breaks!"

Human beings usually resent being compared to machines. But the truth is that we are extraordinarily complex machines. Of course, we have souls and a collection of functional and dysfunctional tonalities that ordinary machines lack. When physical laws are applied, however, machines and humans are indeed similar.

The mechanical aspect of the heart—its pumping action—results from electricity that stimulates the heart muscle to contract. This is generated in a tiny "battery" called the sinus node (about 10 to 20 mm by 5 mm [2/5 to 4/5 in by 1/5 in]). It is the heart's "natural pacemaker." When its charge becomes depleted, the heartbeat slows down and a permanent artificial pacemaker may be needed to provide the heart with an adequate heart rate. When the pump contracts, it ejects blood and generates a pressure that is transmitted throughout the body through a

It is Never Too Late—At Least for Some

Frank, a 77-year-old patient of mine, asked me this question:

"Doc, lately I've been having three orgasms a week, and I feel exhausted. Do you think that sex will rejuvenate me or kill me?"

"I don't know, Frank, that's a close call!"

That was the beginning of a dialogue I had with a very dear patient of mine, an ex-U.S. Marine, a decorated World War II veteran who fought in the jungles of Southeast Asia. During a visit to my office, I noticed that he no longer suffered from insomnia, and the reason was "intense sexual activity." He had gotten involved with a sexually adventurous woman of about his age. Our conversation went on:

"Two months ago, she invited me to her apartment and gave me a cup of coffee. She told me that I didn't look right, that my expression was kind of sad. Two seconds later, she suggested I needed sex, but the type of sex most men love and don't usually get. So, I asked her, like a candid jerk: 'What kind of sex are you talking about?' She answered, 'Drop your pants and you'll find out.'"

"What did you tell her, Frank?"

"Nothing. I was in shock; I didn't know what to say. Even worse, I didn't know what to do. Finally, the movie started...!"

"It sounds like you could rate it XXX."

"That's right. I told her, 'Hey, look, I don't know if I'll be able to do this.'"

"What did she say?"

"'Let's try and see.' So, she began to..."

"You mean..."

"That's exactly what I mean, oral sex, you know? They call it fellotio."

"No, Frank, the right spelling is f-e-l-l-a-t-i-o..."

"Well, whatever you want to call it—she did it."

"Oh, brother..."

"I've been going to her apartment three times a week. That's all she does: No emotions, no hugging, no conversation."

"That's a strange relationship, Frank. Did you ask her why she only does that?

"Yes, she said it keeps her young!

"No kidding?"

"When we are done, she always follows the same routine: she gives me a large glass of orange juice, makes me drink it, slaps my arm, and says, 'Now, you can go. Come back in three days.' I say, 'No, I won't. I'm very tired.' And she tells me, 'Oh yes, you will.' And so far, she's been right. It's like an addiction. I don't know where I've got the strength to do this at my age. I think one of these days I'm going to collapse at her apartment."

"Frank, you have to be careful. This is getting to be dangerous for you. It's physically too demanding. You have some cardiac problems. Your heart might not be able to tolerate it."

"Doc, you're not only my doctor, you're my friend. I'll be honest with you. I lived my life. I'm a sick man. How much longer can I live? I'm alone in this world. What the hell? If I die, I die. And let me tell you this: I'd rather die from oral sex at this woman's apartment than having a cardiac arrest from boredom and loneliness at mine."

"Frank, you made it through World War II in the Pacific. I just hope that you'll survive this battle, too."

system of "tubes" called arteries and veins. The heart contains valves that open and close every second, letting the blood circulate inside the cardiac chambers, and finally allowing the precious fuel to come out of it.

If this performance is not a machine-like operation, I don't know what a machine is. Now, assuming that the cardiovascular system acts like a mechanical device, let's see what parts of this complex structure need regular checkups, tune-ups, and repairs.

The Doctor's Examination

A medical examination requires good communication between patient and doctor. In fact, most of the exam involves listening and talking. The actual physical examination is the shortest part of the process. Next, we'll mention the essential parts of the cardiovascular apparatus, and how a physician assesses them during a physical examination.

- **Carotid arteries.** Are there any blockages in the right carotid artery, the left, or both? And if so, how severe are they?
- **Neck veins.** Are they flat or engorged? In cases of heart failure they are fully distended
- **Heart.** Five structures must be examined:
  - **Heart muscle.** Does it contract normally? Is it weak?
  - **Coronary arteries.** Are they narrowed by atherosclerosis, and if so, to what extent? How serious a threat do they represent?
  - **Valves (aortic, pulmonary, mitral, and tricuspid).** Are they narrowed (valvular stenosis) or do they leak (valvular regurgitation, incompetence or valvular insufficiency)?
  - **Electrical (conducting) system of the heart.** Are there any arrhythmias, blockages, or any other abnormalities of the electrical wiring system?

- **Pericardium.** Is there an abnormal amount of fluid in the pericardial sac?

- **Aorta (thoracic and abdominal).** Is it dilated? Is there an aneurysm? What's the size of it? How often and how closely does it need to be checked?

- **Pulses in the upper and lower extremities.** Are these present or are some missing?

- **Blood pressure.** Is it normal or abnormal? At times, it should be checked in both arms.

- **Pulse.** Is it bounding or weak? Is the pulse rate too slow (bradycardia) or too fast (tachycardia)?

- **Venous disease and edema.** Examination of the lower extremities (varicosities, superficial or deep phlebitis) and assessment of fluid accumulation (edema).

- **Blood tests.** Red and white cell count, chemical profile, serum lipids profile (cholesterol, HDL, LDL, and triglycerides), thyroid profile, C-reactive protein, and so on.

- **Other organs and systems.** Physical examination of other organs and systems as applicable.

- **Special exams.** In select cases, other examinations are necessary to assess eye grounds (retinal examination [fundoscopy]), occlusion of arteries of the gut (intestinal angina), and interrogation of the cerebral circulation.

All the above are screened in one examination. Additional tests may be needed, and could be any of the following: ECG, chest X-ray, echocardiogram, nuclear scans, MRI (magnetic resonance imaging), MRA (magnetic resonance angiogram), EBCT (electron beam computed topography), several types of stress testing (with or without the injection of nuclear substances), ambulatory ECG monitoring (Holter recording), cardiac catheterization, or a coronary angiogram.

In cardiovascular disease, there's what I call "the deceptive gap," namely, the difference between what the patient feels and what the patient has. Critical narrowing of carotid or coronary arteries, severe heart valve abnormalities, or aortic aneurysms that can burst at any time may all be notoriously silent. A patient who has a life-threatening disease may have no symptoms whatsoever. Therefore, it is essential to detect the presence of these silent killers before they fire a deadly bullet. Fortunately, the technology and treatment modalities available today are truly impressive. A physician who suspects a silent but life-threatening condition has an excellent chance of discovering and treating it.

AGING AND CARDIOVASCULAR FUNCTION

Persons over the age of 65 are the fastest-growing segment of the population in the United States and most Western countries. The average life expectancy for a 65-year-old is an additional 16.9 years.

Almost 65 percent of those with hypertension are under 65 years of age, and about 50 percent of persons with heart disease are under that age.

In the United States, for men, prevalence of myocardial infarction is 1 percent at ages 35 to 44 years and 16 percent at age 75 and over. In women, the prevalence is less than 1 percent ages 35 to 44 years and 13 percent at age 75 and over.

Two-thirds of the total health care costs for heart disease are spent on the elderly. This represents $50 billion annually just for acute myocardial infarctions.

The heart, like other organs, cannot escape some degree of natural deterioration. Nevertheless, the heart can go on functioning normally until advanced age, unless coronary artery disease or other abnormalities develop.

The aging cardiac changes consist of scarring of the muscle cells (fibrosis). These generally do not affect the performance of the heart at rest. However, stress due to excessive efforts or disease does. Heart failure is more prevalent in the elderly, as are cardiac arrhythmias (slow, fast, or irregular beatings of the heart).

In the elderly, 20 to 30 percent of cardiac muscle cells become atrophic, and the remaining healthy cells become larger and thicker to compensate for the deficit (hypertrophy). The arterial system becomes stiffer, and that raises blood pressure. This demands extra effort by the heart to push blood forward into the circulation.

Atherosclerotic heart disease also increases with age, and so does the calcification of the aortic and mitral valves and other cardiac structures. Cerebral arteries are also stiffer, and when, for a number of reasons, the blood pressure falls below desirable levels, the pressure inside those cerebral vessels also falls. Then the brain does not receive enough blood, and this may result in dizziness or fainting.

Sexuality in Late Adulthood
One of the myths of our Western culture is the widespread belief that sex is almost the exclusive privilege of the young, healthy, and attractive. Reality shows that the need for excitement, pleasure, and intimacy continues for as long as we live. This does not mean that sexual capacity remains unchanged over the years. There are changes, of course.

Female Sexuality
Aging alone is not responsible for decreased sexual interest or response in women, unless general health is impaired. Postmenopausal changes, which vary in severity among different women, influence the sexual response.

Although breast sensitivity to stimulation continues, there is little or no increase in breast size during sexual arousal. Reduced muscle size and

An Elderly Woman Ready to Marry an Elderly Man:

"Doctor, do you think John is too old for sex?"
"No, Madam, unless you think he's too young."

It was midnight when my patient Jack, who had just turned 84, was taken to the emergency room gasping for air. He had heart failure (pulmonary edema). He had become acutely short of breath "while eating at a restaurant."

As I was driving back home, I remembered his frightened expression, his labored breathing, and his red robe with matching slippers. Suddenly, I realized that something in Jack's story wasn't right: If he had arrived at the emergency room with a red robe and slippers, he couldn't have possibly come directly from a restaurant. On the other hand, if he had returned to his apartment to change his clothes and shoes to wear lighter ones, he couldn't have been so acutely and drastically short of breath, as he described.

Next morning, I visited Jack in the ICU. He looked much better. I asked him: "Jack, there's something I don't understand about the story you told me last night about the incident at a restaurant. I saw you in the emergency room wearing a robe and slippers. You told me you had come to the hospital directly from the restaurant. Jack, nobody goes to a restaurant dressed in a robe and slippers. I'm trying to figure out why you told me you came to the hospital from a restaurant, when in fact, you came from your apartment."

Jack's lips started to shake, and he began acting like a child caught telling a lie.

"Dr. Eduardo," he mumbled. "Please, get closer to me."

"Jack, I'm sorry, I can't get any closer."

"Why?"

"Jack, you have bad breath!"

"Doctor Eduardo, listen to me. I didn't tell you the whole truth…Last night was my wedding night."

"No! Jack, mazeltov!"

"Thank you, thank you!"

"Jack, did you try something sexual and it was too much for you?"

"You're correct!"

"Jack, at your age, it isn't as easy to get an erection as it was 40 years ago."

"Doc, what erections are you talking about? I haven't had one since Mussolini. She came perfumed and wearing a sexy outfit. It was nice, but frankly, it disturbed me. I wanted to do my best. I tried and tried. What an effort that was. Soon, I began to have chest pains, and I couldn't catch my breath. Rescue came right away and took me to the hospital. You know the rest."

"Jack, I'm glad you told me the real story. You'll have to avoid physical efforts for a while. Then, we'll talk about your marital situation again. And I'll have to speak to your wife, too. Jack, as you can see, sometimes lovemaking can be rough."

"Rough? You're not kidding. I hope that nothing similar will ever happen to you."

"I hope that too, Jack. Hey, relax now. I'll see you tomorrow."

strength lead to diminished muscular tension, and this is at least partly responsible for the reduced intensity of orgasms.

Clitoral responsiveness does not decrease with aging, but the vagina is affected in two ways: elasticity decreases and dryness increases. This can be overcome by estrogen treatment (vaginal creams) or by the use of a lubricant, such as K-Y jelly. Shrinkage of vaginal tissues is less pronounced in women who have regular sexual activity.

Male Sexuality

Changes in men are different. For one thing, their reproductive capacity continues with aging. Although sperm production slows after age 40, it continues into the nineties. Testosterone production gradually declines from age 60 on, but the hormonal decline in men isn't as pronounced as in women. Those who sustain a significant drop in testosterone levels —the so-called male climacteric—show easy fatigability, poor appetite, decreased sexual desire, reduced or lost potency, irritability, and concentration difficulties. In such cases, and only when low levels of testosterone are proven, testosterone injections may help. These injections should not be used without prior medical/urological evaluation; under certain circumstances, they may be dangerous. For example, an undiagnosed malignant tumor of the prostate may grow rapidly due to testosterone administration.

The male sexual response is affected by aging in a number of ways. It usually takes a longer time and more direct stimulation of the penis for it to become erect. Erections are generally less firm than at earlier ages. The amount of semen is reduced, as is the intensity of ejaculation. The urge to ejaculate is less pronounced, and the time interval between ejaculations becomes longer.

Lack of understanding or insufficient knowledge about age-related changes in sexuality may lead a person or his or her sexual partner to

High-Altitude Pulmonary Edema and a Fiftieth Wedding Anniversary that Had To Be Celebrated at Sea Level

Sam and Sadie traveled to the Rocky Mountains to celebrate their fiftieth wedding anniversary at an altitude of 9,000 feet. They prepared the champagne, the candlelight, and everything that was pertinent for such a momentous occasion. Sadie felt short of breath the first night and asked her husband to refrain from intense romantic advances.

A day later, even a simple kiss on the cheek was too strenuous. Her breathing became so labored that 911 had to be called. She was hospitalized with fluid in her lungs, but cardiac tests showed a normal heart.

This is a case of so-called high-altitude pulmonary edema. Some people develop shortness of breath after reaching high altitudes and feel as if they are drowning. In fact, in this condition, a good deal of water accumulates acutely in their lungs. The permeability of the pulmonary vessels increases at high altitude and that in turn allows the fluid to fill the lungs' air spaces. The cause of this phenomenon is not completely understood, but we know that it is *not* heart failure. The condition quickly improves when the patient gets down to sea level.

misinterpret facts and expectations. For example, a woman may feel she is no longer attractive because the erections and ejaculations of her mate are delayed, insufficient, or just don't happen. That may not necessarily be the case. A man may be disappointed with himself because he cannot have intercourse twice in one evening.

Learn to be Realistic

A person's sexuality is the prime casualty of unrealistic expectations. As we move further into the senior years, we must concentrate on what we are capable, not incapable, of doing. We should try to achieve what is possible, not impossible.

In addition to normal changes in sexuality during the aging process, age often brings with it physical and psychological problems that may affect sexual performance, including heart disease, diabetes, anemia, cancer, strokes, arthritis, depression, and medication side effects.

Lovemaking is a complex issue. Every person has his or her own way of expressing love. Some are more physical, and others are more spiritual. There are those who are unhappy unless they experience orgasm, and those who are delighted and appreciative of tender kisses and caresses. There are also important non-genital ways of expressing intimacy and experiencing satisfaction in a relationship. Erections and orgasms are certainly beautiful, but so are holding, caressing, kissing, cuddling, touching, and sharing books, lectures, concerts, and traveling.

The healthier your physical and mental condition, the better your chances of achieving sexual gratification. Perhaps more importantly, your ability to adapt to age-related changes will determine, to a considerable extent, the degree of serenity and contentment you will be able to consolidate.

Chapter 3

When Sex is Not Working the Way It Should: Sexual Dysfunction

A person's sexuality is like the moon; there are hidden valleys that no one will ever see.

Sexual dysfunction (SD) may have psychological and/or physical origins. Proper identification of the cause or causes of SD is very important because this knowledge can help treat SD more successfully.

In 1975, sexual health was defined by the World Health Organization as "the integration of somatic, emotional, intellectual, and social aspects in ways that are positively enriching and that will enhance personality, communication, and love."

Whether SD has a psychological or physical origin, the diagnostic and treatment approach must integrate both components. Many patients have several psychological and several physical causes of SD. Social environment, family, tradition, religion, and previous negative personal experiences play extraordinarily important roles.

Sexuality concepts have changed in the industrialized age. The loosening of family bonds, progress in contraception, women's rights, and marriage based on love rather than economics have all had an impact on sexuality. Families used to make marital arrangements, and in many parts of the world, they still do. In Western countries, however, couples generally take an independent view.

Still, many immigrants preserve their original country's religious and social rituals. A doctor brought up and educated in the United States may find it very difficult, if not impossible, to understand other culture's socio-sexual behavioral patterns. The good news is that the United States is a country where there are not only many immigrant patients, but also many immigrant doctors—or descendants of immigrants who are familiar with the language and traditions of their clients.

Sexuality is a universal concern, but the way it is perceived and expressed varies a great deal from culture to culture. Dealing medically with the sexual dysfunction of an ultraliberal individual is one thing. Interviewing an ultra-orthodox or archconservative of any religion is another matter entirely. I'm not only referring to the patient's liberal or conservative identity, but also to the doctor's.

The essential issue is that both patient and doctor establish a rapport and use it to convey their respective messages. A common upbringing and social background, as well as similar life experiences, enhance communication. Let me illustrate this point. I was brought up in an Italian neighborhood and loved every part of it. I understand Italian people very well. I have shared their customs, emotions, songs, and poetry. So, when an Italian raises one finger, I know what he or she wants. When an Italian raises two fingers, I know what he or she means. That's why I can generally establish an emotional and psychological rapport with Italians right away.

Getting back to sexual dysfunction—regardless of a patient's nationality, an SD may translate into frustration, embarrassment, and low self-esteem. Sexuality is an intricate issue. An intercepting cardiac illness doesn't make it any simpler. A cardiac crisis temporarily halts sexual expression because of weakness, fears, and/or the medical need to avoid physical efforts.

Many individuals who suffer from SD blame the cardiac condition for it. The truth is that most patients who were happy with their sexual partners before a cardiac crisis resume their previous level of performance after recuperation. Those who were not as fortunate often attribute the SD to heart disease, when in reality the SD preceded it. For relationships on the rocks, a cardiac condition means another inconvenience, an added burden to an already thick pile of accumulated grievances.

SEXUAL FUNCTION VERSUS SEXUAL BEHAVIOR

HUSBAND: "Sadie, can we have sex again?"

WIFE: "Yes, Sam, just tell me when, how, and why…"

How much concern you give to sexual matters is strictly a personal issue. Sex is as much a priority for some as it is an irrelevance for others. It's you, not the doctor, who decides how vital a role it will play in your life. There are those who feel nothing else makes sense unless they enjoy sex. Others would rather have a beer with a roast beef sandwich and tune in to the football game. The more resourceful may want to do both.

More complex than the sexual act itself is the matter of sexuality. This is a vital aspect of an individual's personality that involves passion, flirtation, seduction, sensuality, and humor. Genes start it all by printing our basic identity. As life goes on, for better or worse, and often for both, we change. Family, society, history—all affect us beyond the reach of our immediate awareness. We are by-products of our ancestry and culture.

Many influences mold our sexual expression—often imperceptibly. Books, movies, television, relationships, upbringing, family values and traditions, religion, and society all print an indelible mark. Sexuality is a complex issue when we enjoy good health. An illness poses new challenges. Physical and mental energies are temporarily drained. Financial concerns and the family's well-being become the focus of attention. During this process, the personality may undergo a metamorphosis, and changes are common. Depression, moodiness, fears, and crying without significant provocation are not unusual.

Sexual stumbling blocks after a cardiac crisis would make one suspect that the two are related. That isn't always the case. In fact, it has been estimated that 50 percent of American couples suffer from some form of sexual dysfunction at one point or another in the course of their relationships—regardless of health.

Sexual dysfunctions that appear following a heart attack, cardiac surgery, or any other cardiac crisis are usually due to generalized fatigue. This is a common occurrence during convalescence from any major illness. It is reasonable to wait up to 3 months after an illness or major surgery before doing an in-depth analysis about the possible origin of sexual dysfunction.

WHAT IS NORMAL SEXUAL FUNCTION?

Normal sexual function consists of four interconnected phases. An individual of either sex who engages in lovemaking is considered normal if he or she experiences attraction (desire), becomes stimulated (arousal), achieves climax (orgasm), and has a feeling of relaxation afterwards (resolution). The successful completion of the cycle depends upon the integration and coordination of these four phases.

The sexual cycle can be distinctly affected during each phase. The desire (also called "libido") to engage in sexual play (phase 1) may be adversely affected by chronic illness, hormonal imbalances, pain, some medications, psychological conflicts, earlier unpleasant sexual experiences, and/or learned negative attitudes toward sex.

Phase 2, the mental and physical excitement stage, can be diminished in women by various causes, which is discussed in detail in Chapter 4. During orgasm or climax (phase 3), men may be affected by problems ranging from decreased intensity of orgasm, premature ejaculation, no ejaculation, retrograde ejaculation (backward flow of semen into the bladder rather than out through the urethra), dry ejaculation (orgasm without ejection of semen), orgasms with a flaccid penis, ejaculation with seepage of semen, and painful ejaculations. Women most commonly encounter decreased intensity of orgasm or have no orgasm. At times, orgasm can be reached only by masturbation or the partner's direct manual stimulation.

With the resolution phase (phase 4), a sense of relaxation and satisfaction follow. The blood pressure, pulse, and respiratory rates—all of which increase during the arousal and orgasmic phases—return to normal. Muscular tension and congestion of the genitals regress. Prolonged congestion may cause uncomfortable testicular sensation, like a heaviness, or abdominal cramps in women. At the completion of this phase, men undergo a period during which a new orgasm is not possible. However, many women are capable of multiple, sequential orgasms.

Let's explore some aspects of sexual dysfunction in the orgasmic phase.

Female Orgasm

Female orgasms that result from clitoris stimulation cannot be distinguished from those resulting from vaginal or breast stimulation.

Some women have a preference for orgasms induced by intercourse, while others prefer masturbatory orgasms. This may at least be in part due to the fact that the woman is not influenced by the style or the tempo of her partner.

Several studies reported that the number of women who experience orgasm regularly during intercourse is 40 to 50 percent.

Inability to have orgasms (anorgasmia) is commonly caused by severe anxiety, anger, repressions, hostility, resentment, distrust, low self-esteem, poor stimulation techniques, inadequate length of stimulation, or insufficient arousal. Lack of privacy, worrying too much about having an orgasm, certain drugs, fear of having another heart attack (or fear that the sexual partner will), as well as incompatibility, all play a crucial role in anorgasmia.

Women who have the most frequent orgasms are not necessarily the happiest, sexually. Some women have the potential ability to have a series of orgasms during intercourse. Men do not have this capacity.

Male Orgasm

Male orgasm and ejaculation are not one process, although in most men orgasm and ejaculation occur simultaneously.

Orgasm relates specifically to the sudden rhythmic muscular contractions in the pelvic region involving the vas deferens (the two tubes that carry sperm), the prostate, and seminal vesicles.

Ejaculation refers to the emission of semen which may occur without orgasm, such as it happens in some neurological disorders.

Orgasm without ejaculation is common in boys before puberty, but can also occur with a diseased prostate, or with the use of certain medications.

Following ejaculation, males enter into a refractory period during which further orgasm is physiologically impossible.

Premature Ejaculation

Intercourse usually lasts 7 to 10 minutes. If a man ejaculates in 4 minutes, and his sexual partner has an orgasm in 3 minutes, there is no conflict because both are satisfied. Imagine the same man with a sexual partner who required 10 minutes of intercourse; he would be considered to have premature ejaculation.

It is important to remember that there is a special chemistry in an intimate relationship that allows for variations in ejaculatory or orgasmic responses that can be defined as "ideal" or "inadequate," not because the timing of these reactions is "premature" or "delayed" but because a person and his/her sexual partner are sexually compatible—or not.

Retrograde Ejaculation

Retrograde ejaculation is an orgasm without the exit of semen through the penis. This condition results from nerve damage in an area called the "bladder neck," which remains closed during normal ejaculations. When this area doesn't shut off at the right time, semen passes backward into the bladder. Extensive operations in the lower abdomen, spinal cord injuries, and some medications can cause this condition. It is diagnosed when a large number of spermatozoa are found in the patient's urine following orgasm.

Erection Failure

Erection failure is common. In the United States, an estimated 30 million men suffer from it. It is also a fact that myocardial infarctions usually occur after age 40, when the frequency of intercourse begins to decline in any case. Age alone decreases erectile power. By age 65, one out of four men has some degree of erectile dysfunction. There is, however, considerable variation among different individuals. Some men in their sixties have very active sex lives, while other men in their early thirties struggle with their erections. Chapter 15 discusses erection failure, or ED, in more detail.

WHAT IS NORMAL SEXUAL BEHAVIOR?

Normal sexual behavior is more difficult to define than normal sexual function. Function equals performance. A dysfunction is easily identified because poor erections or genital pain during intercourse are impossible to ignore. But normal and abnormal sexual behaviors represent a more elusive concept.

Different cultures and individuals have developed their own ideas of what is normal and what is not. The right thing to do for some may be outrageous to others.

Throughout history, different people have adopted opposing views on sexual behavior and ethics. Fifteen centuries ago, St. Augustine despised all sexual relations and described them as dirty and sinful in his *Confessions, Book III.* His condemnation of lust was echoed by many succeeding generations of religious figures and laypeople alike. At the same time St. Augustine was discrediting sex in the Western world, civilizations in the Orient glorified it.

Bias and prejudice continue as predators of normal sexual practices. For many, masturbation is still a sinful act. If you practice fellatio, you can be jailed in some communities in the United States, and some religions state that if you dare to use prophylactics, you are sinning against God.

Some Practical Aspects of Sexual Behavior

Consider the case of a man or a woman who desires sexual intercourse once a week. The sexual partner disagrees and wants intercourse twice a day, six days a week. So, one person wants to have sex once a week, the other wishes to have it 12 times a week. Both are independently satisfied about their respective patterns of sexual response and don't want to change anything. The once-a-week individual doesn't need any more. The 12-times-a-week partner doesn't want any less. Both are within the range of what is considered normal sexual frequency. Consequently, we do not call these people abnormal, but different. And there's no question that they are mismatched in terms of the need for sex. This will cause friction, unless a mutual accommodation is found.

Another situation: One partner is surprised or annoyed to learn that the other has been masturbating. The surprised partner is sarcastic about it. Such a judgment may be unjust, especially if the self-stimulation is the result of a discrepancy in desire.

Disapproving and critical comments about a partner, unless tactfully done, are likely to damage the relationship. This is particularly true in the sexual area. The relevant issue here, as in all variants of sexual play, is that both partners have compatible taste and sensitivity, and try to find ways of pleasing each other. Denying any non-harmful sexual expression may create discouragement and rejection.

With respect to oral–genital sex, for instance, it is not abnormal to dislike it, but it is normal to enjoy it. A husband who wishes to have anal intercourse may be as normal as the wife who refuses it. A significant minority of American couples has incorporated this practice into their sexual repertoire. The AIDS epidemic has made this form of intercourse potentially dangerous, and this technique demands special hygienic precautions. A penis removed from the rectum is greatly contaminated by germs normally present in that area and should not be introduced into the vagina. To do so will cause vaginal and urinary tract infections. The latter occurs because of the closeness of the vaginal opening to the urethra located just above it.

Notwithstanding people's personal taste and preference, and the medical implications of anal intercourse, there is nothing abnormal or depraved about this practice. For some, this form of intercourse has remained distressingly inaccessible, even after many years of marriage. A middle-aged man once told me:

"I have a confession to make. My wife and I have a good marriage. I'm a law-abiding citizen, a man of principles. I wouldn't cheat on her for any reason. I have a beautiful home and lovely children. But I also have a problem; for the past fifteen years, I've wanted to have anal intercourse with my wife. She always refuses and never gives me any reason for the rejection. Every time I approach her, she changes the subject and walks away. That makes me feel embarrassed, humiliated, primitive, and subhuman. So, I decided not to bother her any more. You don't have the vaguest idea about the frustration that I've been going through every night for so many years, being so close to her and not being allowed to do that. I'm not kidding when I tell you that I'd gladly give a few years of my life to satisfy that desire."

Both of these people had normal tendencies: One liked a sexual option and the other didn't. It was fortunate that they had other things in common, which eclipsed their disagreement on that particular issue. In many cases, however, substantial discrepancies in the expression of sexuality become acutely intrusive and upsetting. The couple can face serious trouble, particularly when one sexual partner underestimates the seriousness of the conflict or lacks the necessary knowledge, ability, or willingness to negotiate a compromise.

THE IMPORTANCE OF IDENTIFYING THE CAUSE OF AN SD

Identifying the cause or causes of an SD—that is, whether it is physical or psychological in nature—is critical to treating it. A medical investigation of an SD may disclose an unsuspected illness, such as diabetes, low serum-testosterone levels, thyroid gland abnormalities, a pituitary tumor, anemia, hypertension, pulmonary disease, liver disease, a neurological disorder, depression, vascular or heart disease, and/or side effects from medications.

The more precise the identification of the SD's origin, the more focused and effective treatment can be. Errors can be avoided as well. Consider the following: A man has a penile prosthesis inserted without any preoperative psychological evaluation. He has normal erections, but he is impotent with his wife. He believes that a rigid penis can turn an unhappy marriage into a happy one. So, he has surgery to implant the prosthesis, but his marital relationship remains sour and forces him to divorce. Now, he is stuck with a penile prosthesis that he doesn't need and cannot remove without serious risk of permanent impotence.

The SD Medical Work-Up
- History and physical examination
- Laboratory tests—complete blood count and serum chemical profile
- Serum lipids panel
- Glucose tolerance test (to detect diabetes)
- Thyroid function tests
- Serum free and total testosterone
- Prolactin test (Prolactin is a hormone elevated in patients who have an SD due to a pituitary tumor)
- PSA (prostate-sensitive antigen) test to rule out prostate cancer
- Urine, prostate, and urethral cultures—if there is evidence or history of urinary tract infections
- Nocturnal penile erection monitoring

There is an instrument that monitors penile rigidity during uninterrupted sleep—the Regis Can (Dacomed Corpora, MN). Some specialists prefer using a sleep laboratory when psychogenic impotence is seriously considered (psychogenic implies a mental–emotional disturbance as the cause of impotence). Presence of nocturnal erections with good circumference of the penis and good rigidity highly favors a psychological origin of the SD. Their absence strongly suggests, but does not confirm, a physical cause of the SD.

- Monitoring erection response to visual sex stimulation: A positive reaction favors a psychological cause.
- Pharmacological agent injection testing: A consistent failure to respond to penile vasoactive agents injected into the penis (papaverine, phentolamine, prostaglandin E) is highly indicative of a vascular blockage causing the SD.
- Doppler or sonographic: Evaluation of the penile arteries and the cavernosal tissue helps to determine the adequacy of penile blood flow.
- Other neurological testing: Decreased tactile sensation of the penis or perineum (the area around the anus and genitals) or decreased penile tactile sensation during intercourse suggests a sensory deficit due to nerve damage. Sophisticated penile nerve studies can measure nerve conduction velocity.
- Evaluation of artery patency (degree of obstruction or non-obstruction): To evaluate the patency of the arteries supplying blood to the penis and exclude the possibility of penile venous-occlusive disease (disorder of the veins of the penis), angiography and cavernosometry are done in selected cases.

For evaluation of sexual dysfunction in women, please see Chapter 4.

Comments on Some Basic Laboratory Tests for SD

- **Complete blood count.** The complete blood count may show enough abnormalities to identify the SD as generally physical in origin. Common test results and their associated disorders include low red cell count (anemia), high red cell count (polycythemia), and abnormal white cells (leukemia), among others.

- **Glucose tolerance test.** Exclusion of diabetes is a must in SD detection. In fact, diabetes is often first discovered as part of the work-up for SD.

- **Serum free and total testosterone.** This determination is particularly important in the presence of erectile dysfunction (ED), when the ED is partial and the patient is able to get some rigidity. When the free testosterone is abnormally low, the patient will usually improve with testosterone injections. The testosterone blood levels show daily fluctuations. Total testosterone levels are compared with free testosterone levels: if both are normal, there's no need for further testosterone testing. If one is normal and the other is not, it is reasonable to repeat the tests.

- **Prolactin test.** Some doctors also order serum prolactin levels during the initial laboratory evaluation of an SD—along with tests for serum luteinizing hormone (LH) and follicle-stimulating hormone (FSH) levels—when the pituitary gland is suspected to be the cause of the ED. If serum prolactin levels are increased, a CT scan of the head is indicated to rule out the presence of a prolactin-secreting pituitary tumor.

PHYSICAL CAUSES OF SEXUAL DYSFUNCTION

The six main physical causes for sexual dysfunction in the male cardiac patient are: cardiological, vascular, general medical illnesses, neurological, urological, and drug-related. For female cardiac patients, gynecological causes are added to the list (Chapter 4).

Cardiological

Heart disease, like other illnesses, may produce sexual impairment due to generalized weakness. Chest pains, shortness of breath, palpitations, dizziness, and/or fainting are also limiting factors. If the patient has any of these symptoms, alone or in combination, a medical evaluation is needed before engagement in intercourse.

Aortic Valvular Insufficiency (a leaking aortic valve) Warns a Honeymooner

Fred was a twenty-five-year-old athletic young man who hadn't been feeling well for the past three months. He fatigued easily while playing tennis. Since he was about to get married, he thought his honeymoon at a relaxing resort, along with plenty of rest and lovemaking, would restore his energies. But it didn't. In fact, sexual activity was exhausting. He was also getting increasingly short of breath. His echocardiogram showed severe leakage of the aortic valve, which was congenitally abnormal (bicuspid aortic valve). This was badly affected, and had to be replaced. He recovered well.

Bicuspid aortic valve is the second most common congenital abnormality of the heart. (mitral valve prolapse is the most common). Its incidence in the general population is about two percent; among men, the incidence is 2.5 times higher than among females.

Vascular

This category involves atherosclerotic disease of the arteries that supply blood to the penis. When these become blocked, erection fails. Erections draw anywhere between 6 and 60 times the amount of blood that flows to the penis when it is not erect. Obstruction of the penile arteries often occurs in association with diabetes, high blood cholesterol levels, smoking, and hypertension. Arteries in the pelvic area (lower abdomen) that contribute to genital blood supply can also develop blockages after radiation therapy for cancer of the prostate, extensive operations in the lower abdominal area, and complicated fractures of the pelvic bones.

Diseases of the veins can cause trouble because the blood delivered to the genitals is slowly removed during the erection process. The penis becomes rigid when it is congested with arterial blood, but it keeps the erection when the veins of the penis hold that blood for a while. There are conditions where the venous blood leaks out through venous channels, called "leaks." When the blood is diverted like this, the erection is lost. Many patients who were thought to be impotent in the past due to psychological reasons were later found to have venous leaks. Such seepage can be corrected by surgery. Impotence from blocked arteries may be treated with Viagra or other methods (Chapter 16).

General Medical Illnesses

So many diseases can affect sexual functioning that it is not possible to list them all here. Just to give you a general idea, here are a few examples: headaches, seizure disorders, hormonal imbalances (diseases of the thyroid, adrenal, or pituitary glands), lung disease (asthma, bronchitis, and emphysema), cancer in various organs, sinusitis, chronic inflammatory bowel disease, some forms of severe arthritis, lupus, allergies, and anemia.

Severe Mitral Valve Prolapse in a Male Patient

Lee was a forty-one-year-old man who discovered he had mitral valve prolapse (MVP) at age twenty-five. He had occasional bouts of palpitations, but these were well controlled with medications. He had recently experienced increasing shortness of breath during sexual and other moderate physical activities. One night, however, he felt he couldn't catch his breath and was immediately taken to the hospital. Lee was diagnosed with severe mitral valve prolapse and a ruptured chordae tendineae. He underwent successful valve replacement.

Neurological

Neurological conditions hampering sexual function include: diabetes, neuropathy associated with cancer, pernicious anemia, malnutrition, multiple sclerosis, spinal cord injuries, strokes, nerve damage by radical prostate and/or colon cancer surgery, and many others.

Urological

Prostate inflammations or infections can at times produce painful erections and ejaculations, as well as emission of bloody semen. Inflammation of the testicles is also a temporary but uncomfortable condition. Simple enlargement of the prostate does not affect sexual function, but some operations can correct it. Bladder infections can also be upsetting.

Drug-Related

I'll mention here some of the adverse drug effects in males. For adverse drug effects in females, please see Chapter 4. So many drugs can affect sexual function that it is impossible to list them all here. These drugs can cause disturbances in sexual drive, desire, arousal, and orgasmic sensation.

In men, some medications can also produce retrograde ejaculation. Some of the drugs mentioned are used to treat cardiovascular diseases. Others are aimed at the treatment of extra-cardiac conditions, but are taken by cardiac patients at one time or another.

Whether you think a drug is causing a sexual dysfunction and whether you are right or wrong about that suspicion, never stop taking that medication without the health care provider's specific instruction.

Even when a medication is causing adverse side effects, sexual or otherwise, at times it can not be discontinued abruptly and it needs to be tapered off, something that is generally done in a few days. A classical example of this kind of medication is a beta-blocker (see below).

Antihypertensive medications. Beta-blockers (propanolol, atenolol, and others) are used to treat patients who have angina, cardiac rhythm abnormalities, hypertension, some cardiomyopathies, familial tremors, and migraines. They also protect the heart following an acute myocardial infarction. Frequent side effects are depression and constriction of the bronchial tubes, so they can be hazardous in asthmatic patients (Appendix C). Beta-blockers may also impair libido and potency. The incidence varies a great deal among different medications within this group.

Methyldopa (Aldomet) may cause arousal difficulties in women and decreased sexual desire and erectile power in 10 to 15 percent of men. Side effects (as with many other medications) increase in frequency and severity with higher doses. High doses may lead to orgasmic failure. However, once the drug is discontinued, sexual function is restored in a couple of weeks.

Clonidine has been associated with erectile failure and breast enlargement in men.

Reserpine has also been associated with sexual dysfunction.

Diuretics. Thiazides, chlorthalidone, and bendroflumethiazide rarely cause sexual dysfunction. However, there is one diuretic—spironolactone—that in high doses may significantly affect libido, and at times cause some erectile difficulties. Gynecomastia (breast enlargement) may also develop. Spironolactone has been used for many years, but lately it has become particularly well known because of its usefulness in protecting weak cardiac muscles. So, as with other medications, patients may sometimes have to take chances.

Arterial vasodilators. Hydralazine can induce erectile weakness. Minoxidil, however, can cause penile tumescence (increase erections).

Other medications that lower the blood pressure and are often used to treat hypertension and other conditions (cardiac and otherwise), such as ace-inhibitors (captopril, lisinopril) and calcium channel-blockers (diltiazem, verapamil, nifedipine) are least likely to impair erections.

Digitalis. Long-term use of this cardiac tonic infrequently causes breast enlargement in both sexes. Men have occasional reduced libido and erectile power.

Other medications that may affect sexual function:
- Antidepressants
- Antihistamines
- Anti-inflammatory agents (drugs used for arthritis)
- Cholesterol-lowering agents (statins)
- Drugs used for acid reflux disease (cimetidine, ranitidine, lansoprazol)
- Sedatives and tranquilizers

Hormones

Contrary to what people believe, testosterone injections do not increase sexual desire unless the patient suffers from true testosterone deficiency.

The Heart's Battery Fails to Discharge: Sick Sinus Syndrome, Cardiac Standstill, and Fainting with Total Collapse

Louis was 48 and had always been in excellent health. He was active in various sports for many years, and continued to exercise regularly. He had never smoked, and he had a good diet, good cholesterol, good blood pressure, a good wife—good everything. That is, until a week before I first examined him, when he noted that while just sitting in bed, doing nothing else, he felt so dizzy that he almost passed out.

"Everything blurred for a few seconds," he said. "It was a horrible feeling. I've never had that before."

A few days later, he had a severe dizzy spell while making love. Hours after that, he collapsed while walking the dog. He was immediately transported to a nearby hospital where cardiac monitoring showed long periods—of up to five seconds—without any cardiac beats. His coronary arteries were normal.

Louis's diagnosis was sick sinus syndrome of unknown cause. A malfunction had occurred in the area called "the sinus node," which is located in the right atrium. This area generates the electrical current that travels down to the rest of the heart. In sick sinus syndrome (SSS), the area fails to generate electricity. The sinus node is an elongated mass measuring about 10 to 20 mm long and up to 5 mm thick. It can be affected by viral infections or deficient blood supply from the small artery that feeds it, among many other causes. In this particular patient, the cause was a mystery.

A permanent pacemaker was implanted. This is an electrode placed in a thoracic vein by surgical incision. It is advanced toward the cardiac chamber and connected to a small battery that is installed in the fatty tissue under the collar bone. The pacemaker produces electrical spikes that stimulate the heart muscle every time the heart rate slows down significantly. That results in proper ejection of blood from the left ventricle into the brain and prevents fainting.

41

In fact, the chronic use of unneeded testosterone can cause testicular atrophy. This hormone may also be converted into estrogens and produce gynecomastia (breast enlargement).

Alcohol

Chronic alcoholism in men may lead to "feminization," including breast enlargement, female hip configuration, loss of body hair, and testicular atrophy. Many female alcoholics suffer from diminished sexual desire and disturbances in orgasmic response. Social/sexual behavior is also affected by alcohol. For example, overindulgence by men is a frequent cause of sexual assault on women.

Illicit Drugs

Certain "recreational" drugs have street reputations as sexual stimulants. They supposedly act by relaxing and releasing inhibitions. In reality, these substances have no such sexually enhancing properties.

Some of the effects of smoking marijuana depend upon the personality of the user and the quantity consumed. The drug usually acts by producing distortion of time and the illusion that sexual climax is prolonged to some extent. There is evidence that marijuana users have a higher incidence of decreased sexual desire and potency compared to nonusers. Chronic and heavy marijuana use depresses testosterone levels and at times enlarges male breasts. Decreased sperm counts have also been observed.

Cocaine has been associated with increased sexual urges, prolonged intercourse, and more intense orgasms. In truth, studies on cocaine users report decreased sexual activity, impotence, delayed or premature ejaculation, and analgesia. Cocaine is also known to produce serious cardiac problems (See Appendix B).

However discouraging this discussion of drug side effects has been, the same drugs that can affect your sexual functioning are excellent in many other respects.

Furthermore, most of the time, they do not cause sexual dysfunction. When they do, sexual function usually returns in a short period of time following discontinuation of the drug.

Fear of potential adverse reactions does not justify the avoidance of a drug that offers the patient other tangible advantages.

Psychological Causes of Sexual Dysfunction

- Fear of erection failure★
- Fear of intercourse-induced chest pains, shortness of breath, and heart palpitations
- Fear of serious cardiac complications
- Relationship problems
- Anger
- Boredom
- Disappointment
- Guilt
- Incompatibility
- Jealousy
- Power struggle
- Reduced or lost sexual attraction
- Resentment
- Revenge
- Sexual Personality
- Aversion to sex
- Hypoactive (under-active) sexual desire
- Inhibitions

- Partner's physical or emotional unavailability
- Past traumatic experiences (emotional/psychological from previous relationships and/or from sexual abuse)
- Performance anxiety
- Sexual addiction

DISCREPANCIES BETWEEN SEXUAL PARTNERS

- Discrepancies in sexual preferences (for example, foreplay, sexual positions, verbal or physical expressions during lovemaking, post-intercourse attitude, oral genital sex and/or anal intercourse)
- Excessive stimulation resulting in premature ejaculation*
- Intercourse timing preferences (for example, morning versus evening hours)
- Partner too sexually demanding
- Unrealistic expectations
- Post-cohabitation marriage syndrome
- Inadequate sexual information and skill
- Deficient knowledge of stimulating erotic techniques, various coital positions
- Insufficient lubrication of penis or vagina
- Lack of adequate clitoris or penis stimulation
- Low motivation to learn
- Poor sexual knowledge in general
- Poor sexual skills
- Sexual misinformation
- Genital odor
- Mental disorders
- Major depressive disorder or moderately severe depression

- Other mental disturbances
- Alcohol and substance abuse
- Socioeconomic factors
- Differences in cultural/religious background
- Differences in upbringing, education, family values, personal values
- Family-influenced marriages
- Acute and chronic stress
- Financial hardship
- Dissipated hard-earned savings
- Retirement and reduced income
- Unemployment

    Conditions listed apply to both sexes except for those with asterisk (*)

Most of the preceding psychological causes of sexual dysfunction are self-explanatory. Let me comment on a few specific situations.

Guilt. A man loses his wife of many years after a long battle with cancer and starts a relationship with another woman. He is unable to have erections. He's still overwhelmed with grief and guilt and feels he is disloyal to his deceased wife.

Genital odor. This is something that many prefer not to think or talk about, and that's a big mistake. Even highly educated people have this problem and fail to recognize it. It may be due to certain foods, in which case, a change in diet (more fruits and vegetables) may help. Poor hygiene and cleaning habits are great contributors.

Sexually demanding partner. A sexually demanding partner is scary to normal people. Imagine if you suffer from heart disease. It's a real turn-off.

Post-cohabitation marriage syndrome. Post-cohabitation marriage syndrome is a deficient sexual response that may develop after years

45

of living together in a happy relationship and then finally marrying. The new "legalized" status may create new responsibilities and concerns that lead to a deterioration of sexual communication.

Fears (cardiac complications). Various fears on the part of a cardiac patient and his or her spouse are common and need attention. When exaggerated, they can reach the level of panic (palpitations, chest pains, shortness of breath, light-headedness). None of these symptoms may have anything to do with the heart, but instead be the result of an acute anxiety attack. Your doctor can help you alleviate these symptoms. An evaluation and perhaps some form of stress testing will determine if the heart is stable and capable of tolerating sexual efforts.

Safety concerns during sexual activity are understandable, but unwarranted obsessions will interfere with lovemaking and take away its joy.

Fears (erection failure). There are few things men are more sensitive about than their erections. Any erection failure inevitably brings up the possibility that it might happen again. And when a man convinces himself that he will fail, he often proves to be correct. Men who feel threatened by the prospect of erectile failure can benefit from sensate focus exercises. This approach has been suggested by Masters and Johnson for couples who have problems related to inadequate erections. The technique focuses not on intercourse, but on the rediscovery of pleasure in physical contact, and then in genital touching—without intercourse.

These exercises are particularly useful in convalescent cardiac patients. The purpose is to avoid worrying about penile insertion into the vagina. The male partner (the patient) is trained to induce orgasm in his partner by touching, caressing, oral–genital contact, and so on. Once he brings the woman to orgasm, she can help him reach his orgasm. All of this is accomplished without actual intercourse. In future sessions he will be more secure about the firmness and duration of his erections.

Retirement and reduced income. Retirement and reduced income may also negatively influence sex. People who have enjoyed an energetic working pace for many years may perceive retirement as an introduction to boredom. Added considerations are loss of status and prestige. At home, the spouse may expect more sexual involvement because the retiree now has more time available. This is especially worrisome when that busy wage earner had previously used excessive work as an excuse for poor sex.

Survivors of a cardiac crisis are often faced with budget limitations and uncertainty about their future sexual viability. The family feels the impact of these preoccupations. Anxiety and depressive states may last up to one year. There may be moments of intolerance and irritability for menial reasons, and many opportunities to practice apologetic remarks.

Other situations, such as the caretaker spouse assuming new responsibilities, contribute to this moodiness. Husbands assisting sick wives take on the cleaning and cooking, and women with convalescent husbands

Tachycardia and Severe Palpitations

"When I have palpitations, I feel like my heart is a horse trying to come out of my chest. It's a terrible sensation."

Mary was 21, and had had bouts of palpitations since childhood. But these had never been so severe. Lovemaking triggered some attacks, but others also appeared unpredictably. She underwent electrophysiological testing. Various catheters were positioned inside the cardiac chambers, and the heart's electrical wiring system was evaluated. This revealed the mechanism of Mary's arrhythmias. She had successful catheter-guided, radio-frequency ablation of the area responsible for her tachycardia.

Ablation is the suppression of a localized area inside the cardiac muscle that is responsible for the arrhythmia. This procedure is carried out when the patient has severe tachycardia, not responsive to medications.

may need to find jobs to provide economic support or take on "handy-man" chores they are unprepared for. This reversal of roles requires moti-vation and a period of adjustment.

Overprotection of the patient by a well-meaning mate can also be counterproductive. The convalescent may feel like an invalid when he or she is desperately trying to feel and look stronger.

Legions of men and women who suffer from sexual dysfunction never say a word about it. They keep it to themselves and do not seek any professional counseling. The knowledge of the dysfunction is only shared by the sexual partner, who, for a number of reasons, often doesn't say or do anything either.

If the affected person raises the issue with a view to any possible cor-rective course of action, that means talking about the past, present, and future of the relationship. Engaging the sexual partner in the analysis and necessary consultations and facing the fear that the exploration into the psyche may be more taxing and upsetting than he or she is willing or able to tolerate.

Ultimately, your choices are limited to two options.

Do nothing about the SD and keep the sexual relationship as it is—with all its incessantly orbiting, dysfunctional halos intact.

Do something about it. This takes determination and hard work. It also involves some risks at a personal level and a degree of uncertain-ty about the outcome of the relationship. However, if the effort succeeds, the darkness turns into light, and sadness is replaced by joy. The effort may be worthwhile. On the other hand, if, at the end, things can't be worked out, at least you'll be left with more knowledge, more experi-ence, and more wisdom to deal with the uncharted itineraries and unpredictability of future relationships.

Chapter 4

The Female Perspective

WOMAN TO HER PHYSICIAN: "Doctor, are you taking my chest pains seriously?"

PHYSICIAN: "Of course!... Just assure me that you are serious about them!"

Women have complained for the longest time that physicians do not always take them seriously. Things are gradually changing, but an editorial in the *New England Journal of Medicine* written about a decade ago still holds true today. The writer stated that, "being different from men has meant being less equal for most of the recorded time and throughout most of the world, and that all too often, women have been treated less than equally in social relations, political endeavors, business, education, research and health care."

In the same journal, an article published in February 1999 reported on doctors' reactions to videotaped interviews of eight patients complaining of chest pains. The patients had comparable occupations and medical insurance. The tapes were shown to 720 doctors. The results revealed that 40 percent of the doctors were less likely to refer a black patient than a white patient for cardiac catheterization. The doctors were also less likely to refer a woman than a man for catheterization. The researchers concluded, "the race and sex of the patient independently influence how physicians manage chest pain." It was further concluded that doctor bias "may represent overt prejudice, or more likely, could be the result of subconscious perceptions, rather than deliberate actions or thoughts."

Bias still exists. And the biased individual does not have to be a doctor. It could be the patient's husband.

One evening, I was at the hospital emergency room when a 45-year-old woman walked in complaining of very severe chest pain. Her facial expression showed intense suffering. Her husband and teenage son accompanied her. Both loved her dearly. Yet, their attitude contrasted sharply with that of the patient. They were joking and laughing (not about her, but something else). As soon as she was started on oxygen and an intravenous line, she went into cardiac arrest. Resuscitation efforts were unsuccessful.

When the husband and son were told she was gone, the laughing turned into tears and despair. A while later, I was curious to know why they had displayed such joyfulness when the woman was complaining of excruciating chest pain. Her husband, now a fresh widower, told me: "I feel terrible about this. But you know how women are. They're so emotional. We had an argument, and I thought she was making it up. The idea that she could be having a heart attack never crossed my mind."

Another case: I was called from the emergency room to examine a 55-year-old woman complaining of severe tightness in her chest. Her electrocardiogram (ECG) was normal, but I suspected she was heading for a heart attack and ordered her admission to the intensive care unit. A male nurse, who assisted her in the emergency room, said he "was certain she was suffering from an acute anxiety attack." When I asked him why he didn't take a symptom typical of an acute myocardial infarction seriously, he answered: "Because she's a woman." The patient had a very serious and acute heart attack.

Bias in clinical decisionmaking is based upon the perception that women's complaints are too often "imaginary" or "psychosomatic." Health professionals must be extremely careful before they allow themselves to be influenced by such nonsense. Consider the sobering statistics.

Acute myocardial infarctions are the most frequent cause of death in women in the United States (about 250,000 annually). More than 500,000 women in the U.S. die of cardiovascular disease each year. Heart disease strikes one out of every three women. (Breast cancer develops in one out of every eight women and causes 40,000 deaths annually.) Severe heart failure is twice as common in women as it is in men. Men are at a disadvantage, however, when it comes to age and risk of heart attack. Heart attacks start peaking for women when they are in their sixties.

Men start showing signs of a heart disease about ten years earlier, for reasons as yet poorly understood. The highest risk of coronary artery disease in women is seen in older women and in black women.

Tobacco is the single most important coronary risk factor for women (and men). Over the past several decades, American women's use of cigarettes has not decreased drastically as has occurred among men. Women have more difficulty quitting cigarette use. The frequent gain in weight that commonly occurs following smoking cessation is a discouraging factor for those who are making an effort to stop smoking.

Diabetic women with hypertension have especially high rates of coronary artery disease. Obese women and those who had diabetes during pregnancy are particularly prone to develop diabetes. Aggressive management of hypertension and blood lipid levels in diabetic women is extremely important.

Unrecognized Rheumatic Mitral Stenosis Revealed by Midnight Lovemaking

Nothing was disturbing the blissful rest of the young couple sleeping at home. Charles and Nina had a successful marriage. Although she was never too passionate, and they seldom experienced peaks of great excitement, there were no major problems in their relationship. Sex was important, but not *that* important.

One night turned out to be different. Charles woke up at about 2:00 A.M. feeling aroused, and he began making waves. He reached for the radio at the bedside table and tuned in to a soft-music station. Nina was sleeping, but her husband changed that. She responded, and a lovemaking trip was on its way. Engaging in intense sexual play, he soon heard unusually noisy respiratory sounds coming from his wife. He thought that she was heading for an earthshaking orgasm, the kind she rarely, if ever, had. He felt proud of his masculine prowess and intensified his efforts. Only when Nina (who was unable to talk) scratched his face with her nails to get his attention, did he realize that something was wrong. She was desperately short of breath.

An ambulance took her to the emergency room, where I treated her for acute pulmonary edema (severe fluid accumulation in the lungs due to heart failure). This was due to severe narrowing of the mitral valve orifice called mitral stenosis. She had corrective surgery and recovered.

The mitral valve is located between the left atrium and the left ventricle. When the valve is distorted and calcified due to damage originally caused by rheumatic fever in childhood, it narrows progressively. After 10 to 20 years, symptoms become noticeable.

When the mitral valve opening is tight, blood can't flow easily through it and the pressure in the left atrium increases. This is then transmitted to the lungs, and these fill up with fluid (pulmonary edema).

Shortness of breath and easy fatigability are characteristic symptoms, but until they become acute and intolerable, some patients do not seek medical attention.

> That is precisely what happened to Nina, who had been having these discomforts for several weeks. Had she consulted a doctor, the disorder could have been easily diagnosed by simply listening to the heart with a stethoscope and obtaining an echocardiogram. A life-threatening episode could have been avoided.
>
> Nina and her husband mutually agreed that from that point on, before love making, they would turn the lights on and see the expression on each other's face, to make sure that a similar misunderstanding would never happen again.

Social conditions that in the past solely affected men in terms of risk for heart disease, now also influence women's health. Many more women, including those with young children, participate in the work force, both in traditional occupations (teaching, nursing) as well as occupations that formerly were the domain of men (medicine, law, business, and so on). The stress that these activities demand, the physical and emotional hazards of the work environment, plus smoking and substance abuse, have all been implicated in the increased incidence of cardiovascular disease in women.

WOMEN, DEPRESSION, AND CARDIAC HEALTH

A large body of evidence confirms the fact that depression is a risk factor for coronary heart disease and congestive heart failure. In women, these findings have great significance for several reasons:

- ❤ The incidence of depression is higher in women.
- ❤ Depression is widely prevalent in menopausal women.
- ❤ Coronary heart disease increases after menopause.

Women with coronary heart disease typically have poorer outcomes than do men with the same condition.

Timely management of depression is extremely important. Women with heart disease, as well as their physicians, must be vigilant for signs of depression. The condition requires prompt treatment with antidepressants, behavioral changes, and life-skills training. Selective serotonin uptake inhibitors (SSRIs), such as Prozac, are preferred choices.

FEMALE SEXUAL DYSFUNCTION

The expression of sexuality is the result of multiple influences that constantly interact with each other. Sexual responsiveness depends upon a woman's overall health, including, but not limited to, the neurological, cardiovascular, hormonal, urological, and gynecological systems. Additionally, psychiatric or psychological disturbances, a history of sexual abuse, negative personal experiences, the use of licit or illicit drugs, aging, cultural background, upbringing, individual character, family traditions, and religion may also affect sexual responsiveness.

Finally, the quality of the sexual relationship itself is an important influence. Any negatives in these areas can turn sexual joy into an unpleasant experience.

It is important to make a distinction between poor or inadequate sexual performance and sexual dysfunction. Sometimes, a passive, unmotivated, and deficient sexual interaction results from "lack of chemistry" with the sexual partner. It's crucial to be clear on this point, because recriminations by a disappointed sexual partner may generate undeserved questions about a woman's potential capacity for full sexual expression. The reason for a poor or sub-optimal performance during intimacy may simply be a mismatch. The woman and her mate are just not made for each other. Women who were thought to be frigid by one sexual partner have been described as "the most sensuous and passionate" by another. So, there's a big difference between a "sexual malfunction" and a "sexual dysfunction." A sexual "malfunction" may be the expression of unhappiness and discontent with the sexual partner.

When we describe female sexual dysfunction, then, our focus is primarily on sexual dysfunction within a relationship that is not directly related to mismatched partners, but to other causes. There are four main categories of female sexual dysfunction: desire disorders, arousal disorders, orgasmic disorders, and sexual pain disorders. The possible causes of each, and some solutions, are listed below.

Desire Disorders

Conditions and situations that may adversely affect desire include:

- Alcohol abuse. Needs urgent correction and specialized management.
- Arthritis or compressed nerves of the cervical spine (neck) or thoraco-lumbar spine (mid- and low back); severe disability due to hip or knee degenerative joint disease. Seek orthopedic and/or neurological evaluation.
- Boredom, same routine, same positions. May benefit from reviewing erotic material.
- Breast cancer chemotherapy, gynecologic malignancies (surgical scars, weakening side-effects of cancer drugs).
- Cigarette smoking.
- Depression. Don't let it go too far. See a psychiatrist at an early stage. Various drugs.
- Antidepressants and anti-psychotics; lithium; barbiturates; benzodiazepines.
- Hormonal preparations, including Danazol; contraceptives.
- Hysterectomy (it does not usually have any negative effects on female sexual function. However, some women have impaired sexual responsiveness and decreased sexual interest following

this surgery because they see the operation as a lessening of their femininity).

- Lifestyle factors, including serious preoccupations, career issues, financial hardship, children, stressful job, obligations with parents or other relatives, children with disabilities, dysfunctional personalities of relatives living at home, chronic stress.
- Menopause. Acts by causing hormone-induced mood swings and vaginal atrophy. It usually responds to estrogens.
- Medications, including drugs for heartburn and reflux (histamine H2 receptor blockers), phenytoine, indomethacin, and ketoconazole.
- Relationship problems. Please see Part III.
- Situations that cause personal embarrassment, including colostomy, urinary incontinence, and radical mastectomy. Seek psychiatric or psychological counseling.
- Vascular disease associated with diabetes.

You might find this difficult to believe: Sexologists paid little attention to low sexual desire up until 1977. In the 1980s and 1990s, things suddenly changed, and sexual desire problems became the most commonly reported sexual complaints.

Currently, pharmaceutical companies are strenuously searching for ways to produce a drug to enhance sexual desire. Viagra, Levitra, and Cialis work on erectile dysfunction in men, and there's hope that these drugs will improve the analogous condition in women, namely sexual arousal, which is essentially the engorgement-lubrication response of female sexual excitement. But these drugs are not aphrodisiacs. None of them showed any significant effect on sexual desire.

I mentioned above multiple causes of low sexual desire, but there's one I'd like to relate to you very specially. It is an issue that the doctor generally doesn't know about when he/she treats the patient, and often times, not even the sexual partner is fully aware of it. I am referring to the "sexual desire position" the partners hold in an intimate relationship.

Husband and wife (I'm also referring to any other intimate relationship) often have different degrees of sexual desire, and they adopt their respective positions: "high desire" and "low desire." A significant discrepancy in sexual desire between sexual partners creates problems, attitudes, and arguments, which reflect additional relationship conflicts.

David Snarch, Ph.D, a recognized expert in the field of marital and sex counseling (See *Principles and Practice of Sex Therapy* [S. Leiblum and R. Rosen], pages 17–28) beautifully describes the dynamics of this conflict and tells us that "the partner with the least sexual desire always controls sex," AND, "the low-desire partner not only controls when sex occurs, but the content and the style of sex as well."

There are legions of women who suffer from this "marital imbalance" in silence and carry the burden of their unhappiness for a lifetime. Their husbands don't know it, or pretend they don't know. When heart disease becomes an added burden, it isn't always easy to determine whether heart disease or marital discord is the main cause of the patient's suffering, and the sexual difficulties the couple may endure.

These complex issues should only be addressed by psychotherapists with special knowledge in sexology, and/or sex therapists.

AROUSAL DISORDERS

Female sexual arousal disorder (FSAD) is an abnormal sexual excitement response. It is characterized by a persistent or recurrent inability to attain or to maintain arousal until completion of sexual activity, and adequate lubrication–swelling response of sexual excitement. This phase of the female sexual cycle is similar to the "erection" phase in males.

FSAD may be treated individually or in sessions with the patient's partner. Medical treatments are very infrequently considered for pre-menopausal women. Menopausal patients who are estrogen deficient and have painful intercourse and vaginal dryness may improve with hormone replacement therapy, although sex therapy may also be needed.

When the sexual arousal disorder results from psychological problems, sex therapy is indicated. The specialist will try to neutralize negative thoughts, emotions, and behavior. Other recommended methods include the use of erotic material, sexual skills training, masturbation exercises, and improved communication during intimacy.

The sex therapist may need to evaluate the sexual partner's skill and ability to induce sexual stimulation.

Water-based commercial lubricants are preferable to oil-based lubricants in that they will not damage latex condoms and are less likely to cause infection.

Lubricants containing the antiviral spermicidal nonoxynol-9 are safer but can be irritating to some patients. Additives contained in lubricants can cause local allergic reactions.

Assistance from electrical or battery operated vibrators may be advisable. These come in different shapes and sizes. There are phallic-shaped vibrators, "lipstick"-size models, and "palm of hand" shaped models specially designed for clitoral stimulation.

Postmenopausal women: Genital atrophy is the most common cause of arousal disorders. Estrogen therapy may help, but women vary considerably in their sexual response to estrogen medications. The usual benefit seen with estrogen therapy is the effect on the skin, breasts, and vagina. This improves self-confidence and mood.

There are some limitations to the use of estrogens. See Estrogen Replacement Therapy: Debunking the Myth (page 62).

Testosterone: It has been known for the past 50 years that testosterone is essential for sexual desire and arousal in women. This information, however, has not been used properly. Testosterone levels decrease as the ovarian function decreases during menopause, and more so following hysterectomy or chemotherapy. Patients are not usually aware of this. Testosterone deficiency may also cause a loss of muscle tone, decreased energy level, and genital atrophy not responsive to estrogens.

There is concern that by giving testosterone to a woman, she will become more masculine and that will predispose her to cardiovascular disease. It is true that this hormone mildly decreases the good cholesterol, HDL, but some researchers think that the end result of low-dose testosterone administration would actually have a cardio-protective effect.

Adverse side effects of testosterone, which are uncommon in low dosages prescribed for women, include weight gain, liver abnormalities, enlargement of the clitoris, facial hair, deep voice, and a tendency to baldness.

Women with testosterone deficiency usually require far lower dosages of testosterone than those used for men with testosterone deficiency (women's bodies have only $\frac{1}{20}$ as much testosterone as men).

Testosterone may be administered via oral and sublingual tablets, skin patch, and topical cream. Application of this cream applied to the vulva half an hour to several hours prior to intimacy has been reported by some investigators to enhance sexual desire and arousal.

PDE-5 inhibitors: Viagra, Levitra, and Cialis, theoretically should enhance vaginal engorgement and lubrication, the same way these drugs produce an erection. This is currently under investigation.

Other medications that are under investigation to improve sexual arousal disorders in females include prostaglandin E-1, phentolamine, pentoxifylline, various topical vasodilators ephedrine, psychostimulants, apomorphine, and other drugs.

Eros–CTD: This is the first FDA-approved treatment for sexual dysfunction that consists in a clitoral device (a small pump) with a plastic cup attachment, which fits over the clitoris and neighboring tissues. It acts by suction and simulating the effects of oral sex.

Nerve-sparing surgery: Surgeons are more consistently performing nerve-sparing surgeries that avoid damage to pelvic and other nerves.

Medications that cause arousal disorders include: anticholinergics, antihistamines, antihypertensives, and psychotropic agents (benzodiazepines and antidepressants).

Personality and mental disorders are frequently associated with sexual arousal disorders: phobia, panic, anxiety, depression, bipolar disorder, and psychosis (paranoia, schizophrenia, and so on). All these patients need psychiatric management, although some patients with severe psychiatric illnesses may not be able to tolerate psychosexual therapy or benefit from it.

Orgasmic Disorders

Anorgasmia (lack of orgasmic response) may be caused by sexual inexperience, improper stimulation, incompatibility, psychological inhibition, chronic disease, and medications. Anorgasmia is often responsive to therapy.

Most researchers agree that the brain plays a crucial role in the experience of orgasm. So, psychological factors are very important in most cases. Orgasms are complex reactions affected by anatomical and physical factors, social and religious influences, upbringing, sexual assault, a history of sexual harassment, being sexually touched before puberty, cultural, and interpersonal interactions.

Medications that can cause orgasmic dysfunction include methyldopa, amphetamines and related anorexic drugs (medications to curb the appetite), anti-psychotics, benzodiazepines, antidepressants, narcotics, and trazodone.

Treatments for orgasmic disorders include stimulation by masturbation, including the possible use of a vibrator; Kegel exercises to control contraction and relaxation of the pelvic muscles during high sexual arousal (your gynecologist can teach you these exercises); methods to minimize inhibitions (including music, control of anxiety, or fantasizing); or videos with explicit sex. Those who do not respond should consult a sex therapist.

Sexual Pain Disorders

Dyspareunia is female pain during intercourse. It can be due to superficial or deep-tissue abnormalities, including:

- Atrophic vaginitis. Commonly seen during menopause due to deficient estrogen. Vaginal tissues get dried and penile penetration causes pain and sometimes, low-grade bleeding.
- Bartholinitis (inflammation of the Bartholine glands)
- Clitoral adhesions (scar tissue that results from chronic inflammation)
- Cystitis (bladder infection)
- Episiotomy scars (those resulting from vaginal surgical incision to facilitate delivery)
- Genital herpes
- Post-radiation changes

- Pregnancy and postpartum periods (often associated with a decrease in sexual activity, desire, and responsiveness, which may be prolonged by lactation)
- Rectal and bladder prolapse
- Urethritis (urethral infection)
- Urinary tract infections
- Uterine fibroid tumors
- Uterine prolapse
- Vaginismus (spasm of vaginal muscles)
- Vulvar atrophy
- Vulvar dermatitis (genital skin lesions)

Precise diagnosis and treatment by a gynecologist is essential for most of the above conditions.

ESTROGEN REPLACEMENT THERAPY (ERT): DEBUNKING THE MYTH

ERT recently experienced a radical, unexpected re-evaluation and the news was understandably shocking.

Since Robert Wilson, a gynecologist, published a very successful book entitled *Feminine Forever* in 1996, estrogens have been considered the fountain of youth by millions of women. Dry skin, vaginal dryness, and osteoporosis were thought to be preventable. And that was true. Estrogens were also thought to prevent heart attacks and strokes.

There was a drawback, namely, the increased incidence of uterine cancer that occurred in those women treated with estrogen. The addition of another female hormone, progesterone, neutralized that problem, and everybody seemed to be happy again. That is, until May 31, 2002, when the Data and Safety Monitoring Board for the Women's Health Initiative (WHI) recommended stopping the large research trial of

Alarming Wheezing and Shortness of Breath during Intercourse Due to Semen Allergy

Of all the cases described in this book, this is the only one who was not a patient of mine. A colleague took care of her.

A 30-year-old woman used to develop acute attacks of wheezing and shortness of breath a few minutes following her husband's ejaculations into her vagina. One of these episodes was severe enough to justify a rush to an emergency room. The ER doctor suspected an asthma-like reaction due to semen allergy. That was the correct diagnosis.

The condition is rare and often misdiagnosed. The female genital area may appear red and swollen, and the patient experiences a local burning sensation. These symptoms may last from hours to days. They usually appear within 5 minutes of contact with semen and may also occur within 30 minutes, although there are also delayed reactions.

Allergy to semen is due to any of the multiple proteins found in *all* semen. However, in some cases, it is an *individual's* semen that triggers a reaction. In other words, the sexual partner *may or may not be allergic to another sexual partner's semen.* Oral contact with semen has caused facial acne, but allergic reactions seem less frequent than with vaginal contact.

Female genital inflammatory changes may be confused with monilial infection or sexually transmitted diseases, such as herpes simplex virus type 2.

Semen allergy can be disruptive to interpersonal relationships. The simplest treatment approach is the use of condoms. Some centers, such as the University of Cincinnati, treat the condition by desensitizing the patient with the sexual partner's semen and injections similar to regular allergy shots. The ejaculate large and small proteins are separated. The woman is skin-tested to these proteins to determine which ones she reacts to. She is then desensitized over several hours with injections of these proteins repeated every 10 to 15 minutes at increasing concentrations. The treatment is considered successful if the woman is instilled with her sexual partner's semen into the vagina and she has no symptoms.

women taking estrogen plus progestin (progesterone). Researchers reported an excessive incidence of breast cancer, as well as an increased risk of coronary heart disease, stroke, and pulmonary embolism among women receiving .625 mg of conjugated equine estrogen plus 2.5 mg of medroxyprogesterone acetate, compared with women receiving a placebo.

The absolute excess risk per year in this 10,000-person study was seven more coronary heart disease events, eight more strokes, and eight more invasive breast cancers. So, although the numbers were relatively small, it was decided that the increased risk for these events exceeded the benefits of hormonal therapy, and the study was discontinued after 5.2 years instead of the planned duration of 8.5 years.

This was no small study. It involved 16,000 healthy women, ages 50 to 79, who volunteered for the study on estrogen and progesterone.

Half of these women were randomly assigned to receive the hormone combination, and the other half were given a placebo (a dummy pill containing no medication). Neither the women nor their doctors knew who was taking the active medication. This type of research—called a double-blind, randomized, controlled trial—is the most rigorous and reliable type of investigation scientists can conduct. So, if you're ever going to trust the results of scientific testing, this is it.

Until recently, it was almost considered malpractice not to endorse the use of ERT. Things are obviously changing.

There's still a place for ERT in cases where postmenopausal symptoms are severe. If you go through this midlife transition and ache all over, have to fight back tears even when you don't have an apparent reason, have very dry vaginal tissues that bleed easily with minimal contact, and menopausal discomforts make you feel miserable in general, estrogen replacement therapy can be very useful. What doses and for how long you should be treated is up to you and your doctor.

THE RETURN TO LOVEMAKING

Limitations during the first sexual exchanges that follow a significant cardiac event shorten the accustomed length of time a couple devotes to lovemaking. It is essential, therefore, to be emotionally prepared to act with realistic expectations. The sexual interlude should be not only briefer, but less intense.

For the woman who has suffered a cardiac crisis, resuming sexual activity requires time, patience, and understanding of her own limitations and temporary physical and emotional vulnerability. You should communicate your sexual preferences to your partner during this all-important recovery period. These include the time you need for foreplay, the way you would like it to be done, and the positions you feel comfortable with.

Use imagination, initiative, and explicit instructive material if necessary. Be as specific as possible. Guide your partner through the intimate experience. He wants to please you, but he has to know how. A motivated, loving man will go out of his way to bring you joy. The truth of the matter is that when an intimate relationship is not satisfactory, the heart condition usually has very little to do with the couple's unhappiness. When love prevails, when that powerful force that permanently binds two people and inspires in both of them compassion, empathy, friendship, and total sense of commitment, cardiac disease, if anything, contributes to deepening the intensity of love and the precious spirituality that results from it.

Lovemaking also requires the recovering woman to be sensitive to her partner's needs. This enhances mutual happiness. In planning the return of sexual activity, recollect your husband's "performance style." Some men have difficulties enjoying lovemaking unless they have full intercourse with vaginal penetration—and they are often reluctant to explore alternatives. Other men adjust to sexual changes without blinking. They enjoy being masturbated by their wives, or finding a favorite position that stimulates them to ejaculation without penile–vaginal insertion. Fellatio (oral stimulation of the penis) is a common male favorite, and you may want to consider it if it is pleasurable to you.

A simple conversation about these topics between husband and wife can be enlightening. Many men physically express their sexuality with a short sexual interlude and a quick ejaculation. A woman should refrain from criticizing her husband or lover for acting like this. Men and women do not express sexuality in the same way. Men who need frequent ejaculatory relief may have the most beautiful and deep feelings of love for their sexual partners. These may be just as authentic and sincere as those expressed by males who perform sexually in a more elaborate and "ceremonial" way.

Availability is just as important as ability. Tender, loving care and sensitivity are not easily forgotten. When trying events and moments of despair are shared and overcome, a new phase of reciprocal solidarity reaches a previously unknown dimension.

Serious health problems are among the most challenging couples can experience. Relationships that survive difficult times, however, also have the best chance of being the most durable.

PART TWO

THE RISKS OF SEX

Chapter 5

Instructions for the Cardiac Patient

PATIENT: "Doctor, do you think that having an orgasm is dangerous?

PHYSICIAN: "Possibly, but not nearly as dangerous as not having one!"

No doubt about it: having an acute heart attack is always a matter for concern.

It is the kind of event that reflects our own vulnerability. It is an unexpected event. This makes it more disturbing because, quite often, you're utterly unprepared for it. Its classical symptom—the tightness in the center of the chest—appears at any time, while shopping, working, writing a letter, resting comfortably, combing your hair, or making love.

Many who sustain a serious acute coronary event react with initial denial: "Oh, well; this feels like indigestion. I'll take an antacid and I'll be just fine!" But, in reality, the constrictive pain intensifies, it doesn't go away, and eventually you make the right decision and dial 911.

After the heart crisis is over and during recovery, questions and fears about sexual activity and its safety are inevitable.

Caution is appropriate when your heart is recovering from a recent shake up, and a reasonable degree of concern is understandable and justified. But becoming a victim of excessive fear is quite another matter.

In Chapter 6, I discuss more specifically the risk probabilities of the cardiac patient during the sexual effort. But for now, suffice it to say that, for the vast majority of patients, after a period of recuperation, sex is much safer than generally believed. An aggravating argument with your mother-in-law may be far more taxing to the heart than having sex.

The following instructions carry important messages. If you abide by these recommendations, chances are that your sexual overtures will not land you in a hospital bed, but in your own at home, where you can enjoy the most pleasurable rewards.

OBTAIN YOUR DOCTOR'S OPINION

Advice on when and how to return to sexual activity should come from your doctor. By reading further in this book, you'll obtain the knowledge needed to prompt your doctor's advice, especially if he/she is reticent to give it. You've probably been under the care of several physicians—family doctor, general practitioner or internist, cardiologist, or cardiac surgeon. It's preferable that one of them address the issue. If different professionals make different recommendations, there may be contradictions that create confusion and misinterpretations.

In some hospitals, social workers, physical therapists, and nurses are more involved than physicians in the counseling role. Institutions have their own way of handling such situations. How much is done by the doctors and/or other health professionals is not the essential point. It is important, however, that the patient receive the necessary orientation and the answers to his or her questions.

WATCH FOR SYMPTOMS

The word "symptom" means discomfort as it is felt by the patient. The most characteristic symptom related to heart disease is chest pain or a discomfort usually, but not always, located in the central part of the chest. The pain or discomfort has been variously described as indigestion, aching, burning, constriction, pressure-like heaviness, or tightness. This results from deficient blood supply to the heart muscle and is called "angina" or "angina pectoris." At times, the pain or discomfort may move toward the jaw, the anterior neck or side of it, the ear lobes, the back (behind the shoulders, typically the left one), between the shoulder blades, to the shoulders themselves, or to the arms (generally the left, frequently both arms, and infrequently only the right arm), elbows, wrists, and upper abdomen.

Anginal pains usually last for a few minutes. When they are persistent (longer than 15 minutes) and are associated with shortness of breath, profuse perspiration (diaphoresis), pallor, severe dizziness, fainting, or profound weakness, an acute myocardial infarction must be excluded.

Symptoms that appear to be typical of heart disease may, in fact, express other organs' abnormalities. For example: shortness of breath (dyspnea) can be seen in anxiety or asthma episodes. Chest pains may result from spasms of the esophagus or inflammation of costochondral tissue. This joins the ribs to the sternum. It's like a form of arthritis. These areas are sensitive to deep touch. Fatigue may be due to anemia (low red cell count), an underactive thyroid, or other reasons. A fainting spell may be caused by a drop in blood pressure that has nothing to do with the heart.

There are many other causes of shortness of breath, chest pains, fatigue, and fainting. It's best to describe the complaints to the physician and leave their interpretation to him or her. You describe, the professional makes the diagnosis. Don't try to reverse the roles.

PREVENT EMOTIONAL STRESS

When you are ready for lovemaking, take precautions and avoid upsetting situations—such as discussions with your sexual partner, children knocking at the door, and annoying telephone calls from business associates. Prepare a relaxed atmosphere and make sure you'll have enough time.

Having the right relationship helps, too. The opposite scenario spells trouble. A female patient of mine once told me that she would rather have a tooth pulled without anesthesia than have sex with her husband.

Mental stress increases the heart rate and cardiac contractility, and the heart muscle needs a proportional increase in blood supply. If the coronary arteries are diseased, the needed fuel doesn't get there, and this results in cardiac symptoms, such as angina, or events, such as a heart attack. Even "normal" coronary arteries may suffer from stress-induced spasms leading to acute chest pains and at times, myocardial infarctions.

AVOID EXCESSIVE PHYSICAL DEMANDS

You are trying to reorganize your life. This is not the time to look for challenges or test your sexual potency. Some men act as if they are running a competitive race between their egos and their erections—and at the end of the contest, they're still trying to figure out who the winner is. After a moderate effort, if you've fallen short of the desired results, stop doing what you're doing and relax. It's unwise to persist. Obviously, you need more time to recover. Take it.

During the early rehabilitative period, sexual involvement should mostly focus on displays of affection and understanding, on touching and caressing. Don't place too much emphasis on the genitals. As important as they are, they do not hold a monopoly on lovemaking.

HAVE THE RIGHT TEMPERATURE AND GOOD VENTILATION

A cold environment may constrict coronary arteries and cause chest tightness. Similarly, some individuals are especially sensitive to temperature fluctuations, and triggers such as cold drinks or cold bed sheets should be avoided. Good ventilation is a must. Hot and poorly ventilated rooms lead to excessive perspiration, breathlessness, weakness, and lightheadedness.

REFRAIN FROM SEXUAL ACTIVITY AFTER EATING OR DRINKING HEAVILY

A meal taxes the heart. And so does alcohol. Eat lightly at all times. Wait at least 3 hours after eating before you engage in sexual intercourse. Excessive alcohol is hazardous. It's responsible for a number of heart function abnormalities. Alcohol-induced arrhythmias may not only be uncomfortable—palpitations, shortness of breath—but dangerous.

DO NOT SMOKE

Are you sure you truly know that smoking is an extremely poisonous vice? It causes disability and death. Yet, smokers love it. I equate smoking to having a love affair with the devil. I strongly recommend it for those who enjoyed the inside view of a coffin.

TAKE YOUR PRESCRIBED MEDICATIONS CORRECTLY

Appendix C discusses some of the drugs commonly used by the cardiac patient. Medications prevent palpitations or chest pains, relieve chest discomfort, and control blood pressure. Get to know your medications—their specific purpose (control of palpitations, angina, high blood pressure, and so on), their most significant side effects, and the timing of their maximal effect. Then, apply that knowledge when you plan your sexual activity. For example, sublingual (under the tongue) nitroglycerin's peak effect occurs in 2 minutes and the duration of action lasts 25 minutes. Long-acting nitroglycerin capsules' peak effect occurs in 35 minutes and the duration of action lasts 4 hours.

A nitroglycerin tablet under the tongue, a few minutes before sexual activity, may prevent an angina episode. (For additional information about the effects of nitroglycerin and nitrates, see Appendix C)

If you are taking a diuretic, remember that thiazides work in 30 minutes, and their effects last for 24 hours. Furosemide also starts working in half an hour, but its action lasts for about 4 hours. In general, it is advisable to avoid taking a diuretic during the 30 minutes prior to lovemaking, or you may be urged to empty your bladder during intercourse.

Another word of caution: Don't forget to take your beta-blocker (e.g., atenolol, propranolol, metoprolol) on time. If you don't, you may experience chest discomfort or palpitations.

If you keep in mind details like these, a number of inconveniences can be minimized or avoided altogether.

SEEK MEDICAL ATTENTION WHEN YOU FEEL YOU NEED IT

As much as you don't want to call your doctor for trivialities, you should feel free to ask for help when the occasion demands it. For example, if your anginal discomfort usually lasts 1 to 2 minutes and is relieved by sublingual nitroglycerin, and suddenly, it becomes more intense after lovemaking and lasts longer than expected (say, 12 minutes or longer), and does not respond to nitroglycerin taken two to three times a few minutes apart, you should contact your physician. The same applies to acute shortness of breath, intense fatigue, severe palpitations, fainting, or insomnia following intercourse.

PAY ATTENTION TO YOUR PARTNER

Those shaken by an illness need cooperation and understanding. Nobody questions that. But while the patient gets most of the attention, the spouse's sensitivities are often relegated to a distant second place. Yes, you have suffered a health crisis, but so has your spouse. His or her crisis is of a different nature, but it's still a crisis and may include uncertainties about your future state of health, worries about finances, and concerns about unexpected responsibilities and roles, and so on. Remember: Life disruption is mutual.

There are other concerns as well. Your mate may fear that something ugly may happen to you, especially during intercourse. These fears must be addressed. When the physician indicates that it is safe for you to have sex, your spouse should also be told it is safe.

An exercise stress test without chest pains, undue fatigue, or shortness of breath and without significant electrocardiogram or nuclear scan abnormalities also offers reassurance.

Always keep in mind that you are not alone in the search for pleasure. Often, it isn't so much energy that is required for lovemaking, but rather the desire to please, to be kind, and show goodwill. Use this recuperation time to learn more about your partner's sexual preferences. It may be that after living together for many years, you never asked him or her what these are. Do it now. Misconceptions and intolerance often end in crisis. Promote mutual understanding. This will make the relationship richer and more stable.

BE MINDFUL OF YOUR BODY'S CIRCADIAN RHYTHMS

I don't know where or when I heard that it's advisable to have sex after a good night's sleep. Unquestionably, it's preferable to engage in sexual activity after resting properly. But having intercourse in the morning hours may not be your best alternative. Let me explain.

The word "circadian" relates to phenomena that exhibit a 24-hour periodicity. A circadian rhythm is a daily rhythmic activity cycle based upon 24-hour intervals, and it happens in many organisms. Sleeping patterns, hormone levels, and a number of chemical–cellular reactions in our bodies are naturally programmed in a clock-like fashion.

It has been observed that the incidence of myocardial infarction (heart attack) is highest in the morning hours—specifically, in the first few hours after awakening. This happens with anginal discomforts, too. In fact, even silent episodes of myocardial ischemia (temporary deficiency in blood supply to the heart muscle) are also more frequent during the same hours, as proven by electrocardiographic (ECG) monitoring.

The peak prevalence of these coronary events is between 6:00 A.M. and noon. There is another peak, but less pronounced, in the late afternoon hours, between 6:00 P.M. and 8:00 P.M.

The mechanisms underlying these circadian cardiac rhythms are incompletely understood. There are clues, though, that give us some insight into the problem. In the hours we just mentioned, there is an increase in sympathetic nervous system activity. This means increased secretion of catecholamines (hormones such as adrenaline), which speed up the heart rate and also constrict coronary arteries.

It has also been observed that segments of coronary arteries that contain dysfunctional endothelium (the inner lining of the arteries) tend to show increased vascular tone and constricting tendencies during these time frames.

And that's not all: In the morning hours, platelets have a propensity to agglutinate and stick together. This increases the probability of clot formation. Yet, during the same morning hours, the human body's clot-dissolving mechanisms are lazy, and that certainly doesn't help either.

Incidentally, there's a similar circadian inclination for cerebral infarctions (strokes) as well. There have been other interesting observations. In working populations, there's an increased incidence of myocardial infarctions on Mondays and during the winter months—from January through March.

I think it's a good idea to keep these circadian influences in mind when planning sexual activity. In the meantime, more research is needed on circadian effects on the hearts of patients who have sexual activity during the "vulnerable" hours mentioned earlier. Is it advisable to avoid sexual intercourse between 6:00 A.M. and noon, and between 6:00 P.M. and 8:00 P.M.? I don't know. Is it preferable to choose other hours, when the circadian shadows move away? Perhaps, but we are not sure.

Many coronary events (or strokes) can be prevented or minimized by the timely use of medications that aim at neutralizing vicious circadian intentions: aspirin decreases platelet adhesiveness and clot formation; beta-blockers neutralize the effects of adrenaline cardio-circulatory stimulating action by lowering the blood pressure and heart rate; nitroglycerin (sublingually, in skin patches, or in long-acting nitroglycerin capsules), nitrate-derivatives (isosorbide), ACE inhibitors (captopril, lisinopril), and calcium channel blockers (diltiazem, nifedipine, verapamil) improve coronary blood flow and/or heart function. It's up to your doctor, of course, to recommend the drug or combination of drugs that can assist you and your heart.

HAVE A SENSE OF HUMOR

Keeping your sense of humor during a failed erection or inability to reach orgasm is as difficult as being cheerful during an earthquake.

But try, anyway. There's nothing to be gained by getting discouraged. On the contrary, negative attitudes can only contribute to additional failures. A smile, a little joke, a kind and loving gesture—all can make a world of difference.

When things haven't gone well sexually, put your mind at ease and relax. Read something you like, watch a late-night show or a movie, or listen to your favorite music. If you are fortunate enough to believe in God, pray. Then, go to sleep. You'll see that tomorrow will be another day, and almost certainly, a better one.

Chapter 6

The Right Way and the Risky Way of Having Sex

Awareness of a risk is often more important than the risk itself.

G eneral concepts lead to general conclusions. If we follow that line of reasoning, we may accept the notion that sexual activity is usually safe for the cardiac patient. This is particularly true for those convalescing from heart attacks, coronary bypass surgery, balloon angioplasty and coronary-stent implantation, valve replacement or repair, or patients who have stable angina. These and many other heart conditions allow sex at a low risk. Nevertheless, in reference to your own case, you just can't go by generalities. You need specific, personalized answers.

Cardiac disease instills fear, and fear can delay resumption of sexual activity. Although sex is equivalent to the other modest physical exertions that most cardiac patients perform without difficulties, there are unique situations that require special considerations.

The Framingham Heart Study indicates that a non-diabetic, non-smoker in the general population has one chance in one million of having a heart attack during sexual activity and the one hour following. Patients with cardiovascular disease who pass a stress test have 10 chances in one million. Individuals with angina have a higher risk: 21 chances in one million during sex and the 2 hours following.

This refers to the risk of non-fatal acute myocardial infarction. The risk of stroke or sudden death is not exactly known, but it appears the risk is smaller than that for non-fatal myocardial infarction.

SEXUAL ACTIVITY AND ENERGY EXPENDITURE

The energy spent in physical activities, sex included, can be measured. The technical way to do it is by using a standard measurement called the metabolic equivalent of energy (MET). For example, walking 3 miles per hour is associated with an energy expenditure of 3 METs. Sexual activity is normally associated with an exercise workload of 2 to 4 METs in the pre-orgasmic phase and 3 to 4 METs during orgasm. More intense sex would be associated with an extra 1 to 2 METs.

The average energy expenditure during sexual activity is considered similar to the energy expended playing golf while carrying the clubs, playing doubles tennis, bicycling at 10 miles per hour, or raking leaves. This is just about the energy invested during 10 minutes of walking 3 miles per hour.

Another comparable exertion to that induced by sexual intercourse is walking up two flights of stairs in 10 seconds or several minutes of rapid walking (120 paces per minute).

Sexual Energy Versus other Physical Energy: The Differences

There is a difference between the energy expended during sex and during other activities. Ordinary physical activities, such as walking, are not usually accompanied by emotional components. Sexual activity is. Emotions produce stimulation of the sympathetic nervous system, which increases the secretion of catecholamines, adrenaline and noradrenaline, both of which raise the heart rate and blood pressure in addition to causing rhythm abnormalities.

Significance of Blood Pressure and Heart Rate Changes during Sex

Data obtained from Masters and Johnson's studies during sexual activity suggest that sexual activity may be associated with marked fluctuations in blood pressure of 30 to 100 mm Hg (milligrams of mercury) systolic and 20 to 30 mm Hg diastolic. For example, a pre-coital blood pressure of 169/95 could be raised to 240/120—which is too high.

A study of post-myocardial infarction patients having sexual relations with their own mates in the privacy of their homes showed that the average maximal heart rate during sexual activity corresponding to the phase of orgasm was 117.4 beats per minute (with a range of from 90 to 144 per minute), and the average blood pressure increased to 162/89.

The above reflects the wide range and individual variability of blood pressure and pulse responses during the sexual effort.

RISK ASSESSMENT: CARDIOVASCULAR DISEASE AND SEXUAL ACTIVITY

Before counseling a cardiac patient about his or her sexual activity, a clinical evaluation is indicated to determine the level of risk to the patient. The evaluation includes assessing cardiac status, medical illnesses, mental health, and sexual functioning. It is a global, comprehensive approach. It may sound tedious and complicated to you, but it is not. A good doctor sizes up all these components quickly, assembles the pieces of information, glues them together, and quickly comes up with a recommendation.

Clinical Evaluation

- Cardiac status
- Medical illnesses
- Mental health
- Sexual functioning

Individual Risk Level

- Low risk
- Intermediate risk
- Undetermined risk
- High risk

Definition of Risk Levels

- Low risk: Resumes sexual activity with negligible risk.
- Intermediate risk: Sexual activity is allowed. Carries mild risk.
- Undetermined risk: Patient follows an uncharted course. Degree of risk is unknown. Needs appropriate classification.
- High risk: Sexual activity is to be avoided until cardiac disease is corrected or improved and a new risk status is allocated.

Low-Risk Patient

- Controlled hypertension
- Mild angina (with documented mild atherosclerotic heart disease). Note: I do not consider, as other authors do, "mild angina" a low risk, unless I prove the patient has mild coronary artery disease. The reason is as follows: There are patients who have mild angina and even no angina whatsoever who have critical coronary artery disease. Symptoms of heart disease are commonly absent in patients with critical blockages of coronary and carotid arteries, large abdominal aortic aneurysms that could break at any time and sometimes, aortic valvular disease (severe aortic valve narrowing also called aortic stenosis).
- Mild valvular heart disease
- Past mild congestive heart failure
- Patients with no cardiac symptoms with less than three cardiovascular risk factors—if the three different risk factors are not severe. If a person has a couple of risk factors that are severe, I personally do not consider the patient low risk but of undetermined risk—for example, someone who smoked three packs of cigarettes a day for 40 years, or an individual who

has had chronic, untreated severe blood-lipid abnormalities such as cholesterol levels around 350 mg/dl and triglycerides of about 1,000 mg/dl.

- Post-successful coronary bypass surgery, balloon angioplasty, stenting of
coronary arteries, or cardiac valve replacement
- Uncomplicated past myocardial infarction at least 6 weeks before in a
patient who underwent a cardiological evaluation and was proven to have
limited abnormalities of his coronary arterial tree and good preservation
of his heart muscle function.

Intermediate-Risk Patient

- Moderate past congestive heart failure; currently able to perform regular
activities without adverse cardiac symptoms.
- Moderate stable angina with mild and stable abnormalities by stress testing, and/or moderate coronary artery disease by angiogram.
- Recent acute myocardial infarction (between 2 and 6 weeks before), with
a stable course of recovery, no post-myocardial infarction angina, and
acceptable results from stress testing and/or coronary angiogram.

Undetermined-Risk Patient

- Alcohol binges
- Cocaine or other illicit drug use
- Excessive use of nasal decongestants
- High calcium scores in coronary arteries detected by ultra-fast heart scan-
ning, even in patients without any symptoms of heart disease
- Hypokalemia (low blood potassium levels) or hypomagnesaemia (low
blood magnesium levels), both of which may cause serious arrhythmias
- Multiple coronary and vascular risk factors, even in patients younger than
35 years, particularly in juvenile diabetics, smokers, individuals with severe
stress, and those with severely abnormal serum blood-lipid levels
- Normal coronary arteries associated with coronary artery intermittent
spasms
- Normal ECG with suspicious symptoms of heart disease
- Normal ECG with typical symptoms of heart disease

- Patients of any age who suffer from severe tachycardia
- Patients with murmurs or aortic and/or mitral valve disease, when the degree of valvular involvement is not known
- Pulmonary hypertension (severity to be determined)
- Recent chest pains or discomforts of unknown origin
- Recent syncope (fainting) of unknown origin
- Severe depression
- Severe stress
- Significantly abnormal ECG during a routine physical examination
- Symptoms that may (or may not) be an expression of coronary insufficiency, such as pain in the shoulders, upper back, jaw, ear lobes, arms, elbows, wrists, or abdomen
- Unexplained shortness of breath and fatigue at any age
- Young athlete with palpitations or unexplained chest pains or fainting spells

High-Risk Patient

- Advanced chronic obstructive pulmonary disease (COPD)/ emphysema
- Certain types of congenital heart disease
- High-risk untreated cardiac arrhythmias
- Large thoracic or abdominal aortic aneurysms
- Other severe cardiomyopathies
- Recent congestive heart failure
- Recent stroke. Recent TCIA (transient cerebral ischemic attack)
- Severe carotid artery disease
- Severe obstructive cardiomyopathy
- Severe pulmonary hypertension
- Severe valvular heart disease
- Uncontrolled hypertension
- Unstable angina
- Very recent acute myocardial infarction
- Viagra user when taken with nitroglycerin or nitrate-derivatives

Many of the concepts mentioned in this chapter express personal opinions, views, and conclusions. Distinguished authors have presented "risk stratification" classifications before. While there are some similarities, there are also differences between these schemes and mine. The subject of sexual activity in cardiac patients is evolving. As research on the subject continues, new opinions and approaches will become available.

Chapter 7

The Myths of Masturbation

PHYSICIAN TO HIS PATIENT: "Masturbation, Mr. Jones, is practical, because it's always at hand."

Masturbation is self-stimulation involving some form of direct physical arousal of the genitals—which may or may not end in orgasm. Manual stimulation of a sexual partner is also called masturbation. Generally speaking, however, when we use the term, we are referring to a person's self-stimulation. A few years ago, masturbation received a new name—"Solitary Sexual Behavior" or SSB. This novel terminology upgraded its status and made it more acceptable to rigid mentalities. For example, a strict father in the early part of the twentieth century, upon discovering his son in the act, might have said to a friend, "I found that bastard jerking off." Our contemporary level of sophistication allows for a more genteel, "I caught that SOB doing an SSB."

MASTURBATION THROUGH THE CENTURIES

The Bible's Genesis relates that Er, the son of Judah, marries Tamar, but before she can become pregnant, Er offends the Lord, who kills him. Er's brother, Onan, has to assume the responsibility of fulfilling the Levirate mandates by having sexual intercourse with the dead brother's wife, so she can have a son who will be named Er. Trouble is, Onan resents that an offspring resulting from his intercourse with Tamar will not be considered his. So, he ejaculates on the ground, depriving his dead brother of a descendant. This offends the Lord, who ends Onan's life, too. Because the perpetrator's name was Onan, masturbation is also known as "onanism."

In ancient Egypt, some believed the world was created through God's masturbation, whose semen developed into life. In ancient Greece, SSB wasn't considered a vice, but a safety valve, and there are many comments on this in Greek comedy. Miletus, a wealthy commercial city on the coast of Asia Minor, was the manufacturing and exporting center of a device the Greeks called *olisbos*. Later generations would call them dildos. Imitation penises in ancient Greece were made of wood or padded leather, and were anointed with olive oil before use.

The dildo was used for solitary satisfaction and by homosexual women whom the Greeks called *tribads*. The city of Lesbos was regarded as the heartland of female homosexuality. Lesbos, in fact, was considered more advanced than Athens in the matter of women's education. The island became so famous that the Greeks substituted the word "tribadism" for "lesbian love."

The ancient Chinese were also rather liberal in their sexual attitudes, to the point that anal intercourse and fellatio were quite permissible. Masturbation was condemned, however, but only because throwing semen away was considered wasteful.

BACK IN THE WEST

In 1642, an Italian named Sinibaldi wrote the first book published in Europe about sexuality. He was convinced that masturbation led to gout, constipation, a hunched back, bad breath, and a red nose. Two hundred years later, Ellen White, one of the founders of the Seventh Day Adventists, had a vision that convinced her that masturbation could turn a man into a cripple and an imbecile.

Like the ancient Chinese, the Victorians viewed masturbation as "wasteful," but not for the same utilitarian reasons. In fact, they considered masturbation the ultimate degradation and an unforgivable sin. "Wastefulness" also covered homosexuality and coitus more than once a week.

One of the relatively modern sources responsible for masturbation's terrible reputation was a Swiss doctor, S. Tissot, who practiced medicine during the latter part of the eighteenth century. He thought that masturbation and sexual activity were harmful because "blood would rush to the head, giving very little chance for other tissues to receive any." He insisted that "sex, including marital sex, led to degeneration of the brain, and eventually, insanity."

Tissot's theories had tragic overtones, not merely because he was wrong, but because millions thought he was right. His ideas spread throughout Europe and the American colonies like a virus epidemic. In America, though, Tissot failed to convince the locals that sex for married couples was dangerous. Still, his influence on masturbation's bad reputation for disastrous consequences was significant.

Tissot's exercises in pseudoscientific silliness were not unique or even original. Many individuals, before and after him, excelled in the contribution of similar observations, thus victimizing society in general and their own children in particular.

During the eighteenth and nineteenth centuries, parents and physicians competed in their zeal to "save or cure" youngsters who were thought to have "busy hands." Human imagination was put to work, and

Three Stories about Life Choices

A 45-year-old physician had a heart attack without complications. At the beginning of the second week after his myocardial infarction, we engaged in a conversation about his "future sexual activity." At one point, he said: "I had sexual activity already. I was having erections every night and felt I was going to burst. So, I decided to masturbate…and felt great afterwards!"

A retired 65-year-old male, a college professor suffering from heart disease and diabetes, was "satisfied" with his sex life. This consisted of masturbating once a month. He did not wish to have a sexual partner, because he preferred to avoid "any emotional involvement." He enjoyed his freedom, and because his sexual needs were modest, he didn't see any point in looking for more exciting experiences.

An elderly woman had been married for 56 years to a man who became disabled by an accident soon after their wedding. She dutifully assisted him until the time of his death five decades later. Sexual activity was nonexistent during her married years. She "repressed" her sexuality and "avoided thinking about it" as much as she could. When her husband died, she was 77 and began having "wild, erotic dreams." She realized it was going to be very difficult for her to find a man of comparable age who would be sexually active and powerful enough to satisfy her volcanic desires. So she opted for masturbation and used an electric vibrator. Since she had a pacemaker, she was concerned about possible electrical interference from the vibrator on her pacemaker function. We advised her that with the type of pacemaker she had, it was safe to use the vibrator.

a variety of deterrents were used: belts, cages, locks, straightjackets, wrapping children with cold, wet towels to avoid penile tumescence (erections), tying their hands to bedposts, and inserting their penises into spike-lined tubes.

These were all manifestations of the collective anti-masturbation paranoia. For especially difficult cases, other forms of torture were used. By the mid-1800s, burning the genitals with a hot iron was common; later, electricity was used. Leeches placed on the genitals to suck the blood away, removal of the clitoris, and castration were also widely accepted methods.

It wasn't until 1940 that doctors began teaching other doctors that masturbation did not damage a person's health. The question of psychological consequences remained, but psychiatrists eventually discovered that masturbation did not produce emotional disturbances unless the individual suffered from excessive guilt. Interestingly, in those cases, patients were not advised to stop masturbating but to get rid of the guilt.

Some myths persist, and many still consider masturbation sinful, unnatural, the result of psychological immaturity, and/or harmful to health. Nowadays, even highly educated people continue to think this way.

The fact is that there is now evidence supporting the notion that lack of masturbation may lead to psychosexual problems, such as impotence and orgasmic difficulties. Self-stimulation is currently part of the learning experience in many sex therapy programs.

Masturbation is at times advisable to deal with loneliness, to release tension, and for temporary sexual relief. Sometimes, masturbation is a practical option for post-heart attack or other convalescent cardiac patients who question the survival of their sexual potency. Masturbation may help men by showing them that their erectile power has not vanished and women by evoking a satisfactory response to sexual stimulation.

Masturbation continues to carry with it many misconceptions inherited through the ages, prejudices that follow us like a shadow. Myths are beliefs created by false facts. Never mind if the beliefs are irrational and the facts are based on absurd foundations; Mankind has always managed to make room for them.

CONCLUSION

As far as the effort invested in masturbating and the risk to cardiac patients, it is fair to say that masturbation is probably as safe (or as risky) as sexual intercourse, depending on the patient's cardiac status and the intensity of the effort. Expenditure of energy during masturbation varies. Certainly, there's a difference between 3 minutes and 15 minutes, the pace of stimulation, and the intensity of the fantasies. We are not even sure whether the use of the right hand or the left can make a difference. Is the right hand better than the left? In other words, is one dexterous and the other sinister? If we are going to be scientific about it, I guess every conceivable detail should be taken into consideration.

Chapter 8

Stress and the Heart

A heart under stress can be exceedingly active or deceptively inactive.

Years ago, while making rounds at the University Hospital, I asked a medical student to define "stress." He paused for a moment, and then, he told me: "I don't think I can come up with a precise definition of stress right now, but I'll tell you this—I clearly recognize it when I have it."

I found his comment interesting. The young man, unintentionally, gave me the right answer. He said that he had stress when his mind perceived it. This is an important observation and the essence of what stress is all about—just a perception. So, reality—in a broad sense—doesn't count that much. What really matters is what we make out of it.

Take the example of two Army officers who went to the same war and were exposed to similar experiences. One was badly affected and became disabled with post-traumatic stress disorder (PTSD), a condition common among war veterans. The symptoms of PTSD include depression, anxiety, and, occasionally, violent behavior—all of which may last for years, and often a lifetime. The other officer not only adjusted to what he saw and did in the battlefield, but excelled at it. He ended his career with great promotions and military honors.

It's clear then, that comparable situations are capable of generating very different responses.

Stress is part of life. We feel it even before we are born. Babies inside the womb are exposed to their mothers' alcohol, smoking, cocaine, and other poisons. Many suffer from cardiac, brain, and neurological damage. It must be stressful indeed, to be in such a defenseless posture, unable to respond, scream, or get away.

Life goes on—and not without challenges: children using illegal drugs, teenage suicide (which is at an all-time high), dysfunctional homes, domestic violence, dangerous classmates, serious illnesses and disabilities, financial setbacks, bad jobs or, even worse, unemployment. And then, as if all of that wasn't enough, many have to cope with a collection of personal and family problems caused by unsuccessful relationships.

A prominent American cardiologist, the late Robert S. Eliot, M.D., described in his book *Is It Worth Dying For?* (Bantam Books, 1989) how stress caused by unemployment destroys individuals and families.

In 1967, Eliot was a cardiovascular consultant to the United States government. From 1965 to 1973, the workforce at NASA in Cape Canaveral, Florida, was cut in half—from 30,000 to 14,000. Many of these employees had highly paid jobs. Suddenly, they were dismissed. The consequences were disastrous for many of them; there was an increased incidence of alcoholism, depression, divorces, heart attacks, and sudden death. Some of these victims were as young as 29. At autopsies, Dr Eliot described "literally ruptured muscle heart fibers," caused by the chemicals released into the bloodstream during severe stress.

In the early 1970s, I came across one of these cases. A man in his early forties had been fired by NASA, was unemployed, and suffered a great deal of stress. He was looking for a job. He was a physicist. He couldn't find a position anywhere. Who would give "an ordinary job to a physicist?" he said. He began to have chest pains. When I saw him, he told me, "If I don't find a way of supporting myself soon, I'm going to have a heart attack. I feel it coming. My octogenarian mother is giving me money for regular expenses. Isn't that awful? I've never been so embarrassed in my life."

I never knew what happened to him after that. He and his mother moved out of town and I didn't hear from them again.

Stress has been called a disease of "civilization." Well, that's not entirely true. Cave men also suffered from stress, living in hostile environments, surrounded by dangerous beasts, at times hunting with their bare hands, and then eating like an orangutan, without a fork. Can you imagine? Eating without a fork? And no toothpaste, either. That in itself must have been as stressful as hell.

But the stress of our times is different: Its trademark is *speed*. Almost everything in our society moves *fast*. Indeed, the incidence of heart attacks and our fast living pace go hand in hand. At the beginning of the twentieth century, when life moved more slowly, a doctor treated five acute myocardial infarctions in one year. Nowadays, any busy cardiologist can see that number in one day.

Fast-food chains are also an example of our accelerated lifestyle. They were created to help people have a quick lunch so they could get back to work as fast as they could. But the ultimate symbol of modern speed is the cellular phone. Just a few decades ago, it was fashionable and cool to have one telephone at home for the entire family. Then, phones proliferated and were installed in marital bedrooms, teenagers' bedrooms, kitchens, swimming pool areas, studios, and so on. You name it—almost any space in the house had its own telephone. Lately, the cellular phone has become an extension of the human body. It's used in cars, streets, shopping malls—everywhere. Many use it to make all kinds of business deals from a toilet seat. Who in the world would have predicted 100 years ago that one day society was going to move *that* fast?

Stress can be lethal—and not only for humans. Some animal experiments have been quite revealing. For example, a submissive male tree shrew was introduced to a fighter shrew. The aggressive animal was allowed to attack the peaceful one, but was removed before harm could be done. Separated, but still within view, the two shrews were left to stare at each other. The submissive animal lay still, doing nothing but watching the aggressive shrew. After a few days of intense stress and constant vigilance, the threatened shrew fell into a coma and died.

The hamadryas baboon forms strong, lifelong attachment to its mate. Russian researchers removed male baboons from their mates and placed them a few feet away, in a separate cage, but in full view of their mates. The displaced baboons were forced to observe their long-term mates with new lovers. Unable to change the situation, some of them developed cardiac disease within a six-month period, others had heart attacks, and still others died of sudden cardiac deaths.

DEFINING STRESS

Stress is our physical and mental response to the demands made on us by outside events, people, or our own minds—as we perceive those demands. The capacity to handle stress is called *control*. Stressful thoughts and events are called *demands*. The more control you have over the demands, the less stress you'll experience. Either you control events, or they control you. If you manage to brush the provocation aside, the stress won't get to you, and you will succeed in taming it. However, when you can't control stress, you may suffer from *circuit overload* and react with some of the following symptoms:

- ❤ **Physical:** tension headaches, frigidity, impotence, heart attacks, aggravation of chest pains (angina) due to disease of the coronary arteries, coronary artery spasms (even in the so-called "normal coronary arteries"), cardiac arrest, serious cardiac rhythm disorders (at times expressed by palpitations), cholesterol elevations, hypertension, strokes, physical and mental exhaustion, dizziness, weight gain or loss, peptic ulcer, irritable bowel syndrome (diarrhea and frequent exacerbation of bloating and abdominal pain and distention), asthma attacks, insomnia, muscular pains and spasm (neck, shoulder, back, legs, temples), and leg cramps.
- ❤ **Emotional:** fear, anger, irritability, loss of self-esteem, sadness, insecurity, suspiciousness, denial, anxiety, depression, excessive argumentation, and impatience.
- ❤ **Cognitive:** memory impairment, loss of concentration, episodes of confusion, and impaired judgment.
- ❤ **Behavioral:** alcoholism, smoking, illicit drugs, painkillers, tranquilizers, abuse of self-administered medications (aspirin, Tylenol, ibuprofen, appetite suppressants), gambling, and inappropriate sexual behavior (cheating, promiscuity).

In the United States, the estimated annual economic toll of stress-related illnesses exceeds $200 billion.

THE BODY'S RESPONSE TO STRESS

Stress induces nervous, endocrine (hormones), and cardiovascular system reactions. The brain is the first organ that perceives stress, and it originates the first set of reactions. In a way, it acts like a commander who is in charge of two armies; one, the voluntary nervous system, and two, the involuntary nervous system, also called the autonomic system.

The voluntary nervous system controls the voluntary muscles of the body. For instance, if you notice that a brick is about to fall on your head, you immediately move the voluntary muscles of the legs to avoid it and jump out of the way. We call these "voluntary muscles" because they obey you. When you order them to move, they do.

The autonomic (or involuntary) nervous system is different. It deals with the function of every organ and gland in the body. It has two components: a) the sympathetic nervous system, and b) the parasympathetic nervous system. These oversee functions that cannot be controlled by your brain—for example, perspiration, dilatation of pupils, bowel contractility, and so on.

During stress, the endocrine system (pituitary, thyroid, and adrenal glands) produces a number of hormones. One of them is adrenaline, which raises the pulse and the blood pressure and constricts the coronary arteries. If these are healthy, usually the heart accepts the challenge without consequences. If the coronary arteries are diseased, the heart will respond with cardiac arrhythmias, heart failure, angina, or a heart attack.

STRESS REACTIONS

There are two types of stress reactions: acute and chronic. Acute stress involves "the fight or flight" reaction and makes you choose one or the other. Chronic stress is characterized by vigilance. It is a more long-term state of distress, or a prolonged repressive situation.

There are times when stress can be very helpful. Successful musicians, comedians, and athletes know how to channel their stage fright and fear and give excellent performances.

Downhill Cardiac Course Hastened by a Failed Escapade

Nothing frustrates us more than being unable to finish something we should have never started in the first place.

Henry was 76. He was depressed, and his episodes of chest tightness were getting more frequent and severe.

Here is the story of a man who was described by his family as the best father and husband anyone could ask for, and yet, by the end of his life, something went terribly wrong.

He had been married for 52 years. He was the patriarch of the family, a revered figure, beloved and respected. One day, his wife left Florida to visit relatives. He stayed alone in his apartment. A woman of about 65, who lived at the same condominium, asked him to join her in a sexual adventure. At first he hesitated, but finally, the woman's insistence prevailed.

They met at her apartment. Twenty minutes and two drinks later, the woman swiftly stripped him of his pants and underwear. He found himself bewildered, tempted, worried, and remorseful.

Henry realized that he was in the wrong place at the wrong time and told the woman, "I'm sorry, I can't go on." To which she answered: "Go to hell! You, miserable bastard, get out of my sight!" and pushed him out. He returned to his apartment, crying uncontrollably.

As terrible as all of that was, the worst was still to come. The angry woman turned out to be vindictive, and quickly spread the details of their encounter through the entire apartment building. Upon returning from her trip, Henry's wife and family almost immediately learned of the incident.

Feeling he had lost his patriarchal role, influence, honor, and reputation, Henry developed severe depression and reported no interest in living. His wife and the rest of the family were very supportive. They did whatever they could to show him understanding and forgiveness. But to no avail,

> his cardiac condition deteriorated rapidly, and a few months later, he passed away.
>
> What originally had been intended as a trivial adventure, perhaps the satisfaction of a curiosity more than anything else, had turned into a dreadful nightmare.
>
> There is a price we almost invariably pay for the mistakes we make. Henry's, unfortunately, was just too high.

Other individuals freeze up at the "moment of truth," disconnect their minds from reality, and even forget who they are. During my first year at medical school, a student suffered from so much stress that when he faced a professor for a final anatomy examination, he was asked his name for simple identification purposes and... he forgot it. He kept on telling the examiner: "I'm sorry, sir, I'm sorry. I just can't remember my name." Poor Pepe. When he remembered his name, he decided he wasn't fit for the stressful demands of a medical career.

Following are conditions associated with chronic stress.

Personality Traits and the Development of Heart Disease

Type A individuals are characterized by a sense of urgency, explosive speech patterns, anger, hostility, and competitiveness. A typical example: the successful top-level male executive. Initial studies suggested that the type A behavioral pattern represented a significant risk for cardiovascular disease. Subsequent research could not confirm these observations. It seems that *hostility* is the toxic component of the type A personality (or other types of personality) that is responsible for increased risk of cardiovascular disorders.

Social Isolation

Chronic loneliness is a form of stress. In fact, there is a twofold higher recurrence rate of myocardial infarctions among patients who live alone, as compared with those who live with another person. Emotional support is very important to good health. When loneliness makes its mark, those who don't have somebody caring for them may tend to eat the wrong food, drink or smoke indiscriminately, and miss taking their prescribed medications.

Low Socioeconomic Status
People who have a low socioeconomic profile and poor education suffer a higher rate of recurrent heart attacks.

Depression
Depression is often a response to chronic stress, and is a major contributor to coronary artery disease. This is a critical issue because public health officials predict that by 2025, the second leading cause of medical disability on Earth will be clinical depression. Fortunately, today's scientists have a greater understanding of the brain chemistry involved in depression, and more effective drugs with fewer side effects are being developed.

Experts estimate that 20 to 40 percent of patients with coronary artery disease also have depressive disorders. Depression increases cardiac mortality in healthy individuals as well as heart patients. *Untreated* depression worsens the outcome in coronary heart disease. Recent studies suggest that even mild depression after a heart attack increases the incidence of fatal outcomes.

When the brain first perceives stress, the hypothalamus secretes a substance called corticotropin-releasing factor, which moves through specialized blood vessels to the pituitary—a tiny gland at the top of the brain. The pituitary in turn produces adrenocorticotropic hormone, which travels through the bloodstream to the adrenal glands. These glands manufacture cortisol and adrenaline.

Cortisol has multiple essential functions; it replenishes energy, makes us more active, protects our immune reactions, and converts food into fats or glycogen. An excess of cortisol is detrimental, however. One of the negative consequences of too much cortisol is an increase in the platelet adhesiveness that promotes blood clot formation. As far as adrenaline excess, it causes tachycardia and high blood pressure, both of which can cause vascular damage.

All of the above reactions occur in depression. Contrary to what many people believe, sometimes depressed patients are in a constant state of hyper-arousal and hyper-excitement. This means they experience the increased secretion of cortisol and adrenaline that we've just discussed. In fact, excessive production of both cortisol and adrenaline, characteristic of many depressive states, is thought to be responsible for the development of atherosclerosis and its progression.

Beta-blockers help blunt the hyper-arousal state but may aggravate depression. Meditation is useful in reducing hyperexcitable states without causing depression.

The unfortunate reality is that a large percentage of depressed patients with heart disease receive no treatment for the depressive condition. This needs to change. The treatment of anxiety and depression must be aggressive—as aggressive as the treatment for hypertension, cholesterol abnormalities, and other significant cardiovascular risk factors.

Among the available antidepressants, the selective serotonin reuptake inhibitors (SSRIs), such as Prozac, have been considered the better choice for patients with heart disease, given their limited cardiotoxicity and lower association with weight gain. On the other hand, loss of libido, delayed ejaculation, and orgasmic failure may occur with the use of SSRIs and other antidepressants as well. Different dosages may have to be tried before a medication is successful and side effects are minimized.

Over-Reactivity

Some people who suffer stress are "hot reactors." This means that excitement will evoke a quick response from them that, among other things, will raise their blood pressure and heart rate. In the end, these reactions cause cardiovascular damage. These patients can be trained in various psychological techniques to control their reactions. Anti-anxiety medications are often helpful. Radical changes in lifestyle or life situations may be required.

HOW TO CONTROL STRESS

This is one of the most compelling questions our culture faces today.

A Cheap Pen Can Turn a Life into a Tragedy

Jeanette was a 53-year-old woman who was vacationing in Miami. One afternoon, she went shopping. All of a sudden, her arm was grabbed by a security guard who accused her of stealing a pen. She was taken to the county jail. Her husband got her released on bail. By midnight, she developed a massive myocardial infarction. She survived. A coronary angiogram showed "normal" coronary arteries.

The likely explanation for her acute heart attack is that she sustained a prolonged constriction of a major coronary artery caused by the intensity of the acute stress.

Stress control is rarely, if ever, an instantaneous happening. You don't wake up one day and say: "Goodbye, stress, I'll never see you again." Rather, controlling stress successfully is the result of methodical work—learning tension-taming techniques, including patience and flexibility, and modifying thoughts, feelings, views, and attitudes. This takes some time, but the results can be rewarding. If you are unable to control your stress reactions completely, you can at least reduce their intensity.

Here are a few helpful hints.

- Accept the fact that sometimes it's better to be alone than with the wrong friend, spouse, or lover.
- Aim for flexibility in your commitments.
- Allow yourself to express negative feelings.
- Consider changing an unfulfilling job to a more gratifying one.
- Cultivate very good friendships. If you lose a good friend, try to find another one.
- Do only one thing at a time.
- Don't be a perfectionist.
- Don't eat your heart out with hostility and anger. Focus on positive thoughts.
- Don't fret about things you cannot change.
- Don't try to control other people's behavior.
- Find ways to minimize the pressure of schedules and deadlines.
- Find more time to do what you want.
- Improve personal relationships.
- Take breaks at your job a couple of times a day—and relax.
- Try to turn negative feelings into positive ones.

There are many methods to cope with stress, such as physical exercise, yoga, meditation, deep breathing, a healthier lifestyle, religious faith, biofeedback, mental relaxation, and a very good therapist.

Stress control techniques do not work for all people the same way. Besides, a good method that helped you once may be useless at another time. So explore different options.

Chapter 9

Extramarital Affairs and the Adrenaline Surge

WIFE: "Frank, were you ever unfaithful to me?"

HUSBAND: "Are you referring to my soul or my body?"

Extramarital affairs are common occurrences. At times, they are brief and largely inconsequential. Not infrequently, they court disaster—and when the situation spins out of control, they lead to it. Many women and men get involved in relationships of this kind. They do so for a number of reasons: marital unhappiness, insecurity about their physical attractiveness, and/or the need to prove to themselves that they are sexually skillful.

Regardless of the causes or motivations that lead to extramarital affairs, the fact remains that these often represent a mixture of fear of being discovered, fear of an unexpected and uncontrolled emotional reaction by the lover, or fear of family disruption, loss of reputation, loss of an essential job, fear of divorce, and potential financial chaos. All of these are worrisome even for those who enjoy good health. Imagine how a patient who suffers from heart disease could react to such a degree of uncertainty. Where is the connection between this degree of uncertainty and the possibility of associated cardiac symptoms and/or events? The answer is *stress*. Stress may contribute to unstable angina (coronary insufficiency), cardiac rhythm disturbances, including malignant tachycardias, high cholesterol blood levels, hypertension, and myocardial infarctions. (Chapter 8).

Risks of an Affair in the Hotel Room

Since illicit liaisons normally take place in hotel or motel rooms, not the home the partners are familiar with, special risks arise for the cardiac patient, who is unquestionably more vulnerable.

In these situations, risks are increased when:

- There is a sizable age difference.
- People want to prove their sexual prowess.
- Symptoms that appear during intercourse, which are ordinarily controllable by pausing or medications (e.g., a nitroglycerin tablet under the tongue) are ignored. Personal pride at times forces an individual to stoically tolerate chest pains beyond acceptable limits.
- There is added stress because of the fear of being discovered, feelings of guilt, and/or time constraints.
- Excessive stimulation and excitement accompany these encounters, particularly when they are outside of the individual's usual repertoire, or the sexual partner is too demanding.
- The patient forgot to take his or her medications due to haste and distraction.
- Eating and drinking prior to intimacy have been excessive. This is a frequent situation seen with affairs in hotel rooms.

DOES THE PLEASURE JUSTIFY THE PAIN?

Resentment may also trigger an affair, which then becomes a vendetta, a way of getting even. A 45-year-old woman was married to a man that victimized her and their four children with domestic violence. She found revenge and consolation with a lover.

In another instance, a woman in her forties had a perforated gut due to diverticulitis (inflamed pockets in the colon) and required a colostomy. This surgical procedure connects the bowel to a plastic bag through an opening in the abdominal wall. The flow of feces from the intestines into the bag can't be controlled. When she and her husband were intimate, and he saw stools filling the bag, he verbalized his distaste and made faces. She felt degraded and humiliated. The colostomy was closed 4 months later, and she went back to normal living. But she refused to have sex with her husband again. Instead, she had several love affairs to punish him.

One day, I asked her why she didn't divorce him. The answer was that revenge gave her tremendous gratification. She just wanted to cheat on him, and, she said, "You can't cheat on an ex-husband. You've got to be married to do that."

A discrepancy in sexual needs may also be the spark that ignites the hidden dynamite in an unhappy relationship. If one spouse wants intercourse two times a day and the other likes to have it twice a month, the forecast will be stormy weather in the bedroom.

Extramarital affairs may last from 60 minutes to a lifetime. A famous musician–composer of Argentina in his early thirties married a young teacher. They lived in a handsome mansion in Buenos Aires. The couple had several children. Soon after their wedding, he became involved with another woman. His wife knew about it, but for reasons that were never known, even to her closest friends, she accepted her husband's affair and did nothing to stop it.

The trio lived parallel lives. The composer would sleep at his mistress's house three to four nights a week, and spend the other evenings

Premature Sexual Activity Following an Acute Myocardial Infarction

Stubbornness: Prelude to irrationality

Nothing appeared to be out of the ordinary that evening in a Miami Beach restaurant. All of a sudden, the splashing sound of a face falling into a bowl of soup caused a commotion. A 68-year-old diner named David collapsed into his Boston clam chowder. After an onlooker revived him, an emergency team arrived and took him to the hospital. His medical history was negative except for hypertension, which he had neglected to treat for many years. He was quite a character, however. His wife, who happened to be my patient for many years, described him as "viciously stubborn, easily excitable, bad- tempered, and with a fondness for young women."

David sustained a massive myocardial infarction, which was complicated by life-threatening cardiac rhythm disturbances and heart failure. But his condition stabilized, and after a week in the intensive care unit, he was transferred to a monitored unit. He displayed a terrible disposition toward the hospital personnel, and openly resented nurses and doctors. He did not believe he had sustained a heart attack, much less a very serious one. He had not had any chest pains, so he screamed: "How can anyone have a heart attack without having chest pains?"

He was told that sometimes myocardial infarctions occur without chest pains, but he brushed the explanation aside with a disdainful gesture. He knew better.

The day he left the ICU, he was visited by a "very young, crazy-looking girl," as a nurse reported to me. By 11:00 A.M., David had left the hospital against medical advice. No one could change his mind. When told that his decision could cost him his life, he snapped back, "That's my business."

That afternoon, his concerned wife came to my office. She had learned that a young woman had picked up her husband at the hospital. Though indignant, she admitted she wasn't surprised. She then asked me for suggestions on what to do. I recommended that she start arranging for his funeral. She looked at me with astonishment and disbelief. I said to her, "Sarah, your husband had a major heart attack just a few days ago, and all things considered, he was doing fairly well. Now, if he is going to have sex with a young, obviously irresponsible woman, I'm convinced he won't survive that. I'm sorry to be so blunt, but that's the way I honestly feel about it."

A while later, I received a phone call from the police department. David was found dead in a motel room. Identification was easy; he still had on his hospital bracelet with his name and mine on it. A woman in her twenties was seen running away from the scene. The remnants of dinner and an empty bottle of wine littered the motel table. David could have survived his heart attack, had he not indulged in grotesque excesses. He wasn't a victim of sex, but of his own character.

In 1963, M. Ueno, a Japanese pathologist, published an article entitled "The So-Called Coital Death." He studied the autopsies of 34 coital sudden-death victims during a 4-year period. Interestingly, 25 of those deaths took place in hotel rooms, an additional 5 happened outside the home, and, in most cases, the deaths occurred during extramarital affairs. Moreover, all the victims had alcohol levels close to or within the range of intoxication, and their sexual partner was an average of 18 years younger.

at home. When he died of cancer at 70, the funeral was held at his house. (Several decades ago, when this story occurred, funerals in Argentina were usually carried out at the deceased's house.) And here comes the interesting part: His wife and mistress were *both* present. Both cried for him, both wore black dresses appropriate for the occasion, and each had special quarters where they separately received sympathy and condolences from friends and acquaintances. So, the double life went on postmortem.

Now, don't think for a moment that this was common or socially accepted behavior. Social rules were conservative and recriminations abounded. These came from their own children, close and distant rela-tives, friends, and outsiders. The extramarital relationship, however, not only survived, but lasted until the day the musician played the notes of his last breath.

Such experiences are not unique. Take the case of Carl Jung, a renowned and influential psychiatrist who was Sigmund Freud's close friend—and then became his bitter adversary. Jung was married to Emma, but thought he was entitled to have mistresses. He had a very important affair with Sabina Speilrein, a girl of Jewish–Russian origin, who he had analyzed for several years. Since the psychoanalytic move-ment was in its early stage in Europe, the ethics and professionalism of its leaders mattered a great deal. Since Jung was one of those leaders, he felt obliged to explain his behavior to Freud. And explain it he did. In a let-ter to Dr. Freud, he alleged he had done nothing wrong. True, he "had had an intimate relationship with Sabina," and yes, he "had analyzed her," but he "hadn't been at fault" because he "had not charged her any fees."

Jung always tried to conceal this relationship from his wife, Emma. After years of passionate lovemaking, Sabina realized that Professor Jung wasn't going to leave his wife, and the affair ended. She married, had two daughters, and went back to Russia. It proved to be an unlucky move. Sabina and her girls became World War II casualties. German soldiers shot them in 1942.

When Jung became involved with Toni Wolff, his longest and most significant extramarital relationship, he made no effort to hide his involvement. In fact, he did exactly the opposite. He forced his wife and children to accept her. The explanation Jung provided to his family to justify his decision was that he had become involved with Toni for the sake of his children. He knew, "from personal experience," that a daugh-

Motel Parking Lots Can Be Hazardous to Your Health

A joke is a joke until reality gets in its way.

There are many motels in Miami's traditional and well-known Calle Ocho. One of my patients, a married man just shy of 50, checked into one of them with his girlfriend. He "had a very good time," but when the couple left the room and walked toward his car in the parking lot, he saw a note on the windshield that read in Spanish: *"Te vi, cabron, y se lo contare a tu esposa."* Translation: "I saw you, bastard, and I'm gonna tell your wife."

The man broke into a cold sweat on the spot, felt nauseous, dizzy, and had a constriction in his chest. He was so nervous that he swallowed his nitroglycerin tablet instead of placing it under his tongue. He slept badly that night, and the next morning he requested an appointment with me because of recurrent chest tightness.

A week later, a "friend" told him he had written the note to play a joke. He told his pal that he did not appreciate that kind of joke, to which the guy responded: "What's the matter with you, man? Have you lost your sense of humor?"

The reality was that this man never intended to tell my patient's wife anything. He well understood such situations. He himself had spent a few hours at the same motel, having an affair of his own.

ter suffers when her father does not fulfill his erotic life, and that would inhibit the daughter's psychosexual development. His wife, Emma, and Toni eventually became analysts, followed Jung's psychological methods, published scientific papers, and even analyzed each other. This love triangle lasted for more than 30 years. At the end, Toni Wolff became frustrated and rebelled. She wanted to marry Jung, but he made it clear that he was not going to abandon his wife, despite the fact that he described his marriage as "a brutal reality."

Toni became depressed, heartbroken, drank excessively, and died in 1953 when she was 64. Emma died 2 years later. Jung carved two stone tablets as memorials, to signify what each woman had meant to him. For his wife, Emma, he wrote: "She was the foundation of my house." Toni's stone read: "She was the fragrance of my house."

Some psychotherapists feel that, in selected cases, an extramarital relationship is justified when the couple suffers from "incurable" sexual discrepancies, but have many other things in common—such as children, a successful business association, or a close friendship.

You may or may not agree with this approach to the treatment of marital conflicts, but what I want to point out is that people and psychotherapists have divergent opinions and methods to deal with such problems. Having said that, I believe a physician has no right to impose his or her own set of values on any patient's moral or ethical standards. Doctors are called to help, not to judge.

THE EXTRAMARITAL AFFAIR: ITS DEVELOPMENT AND STAGES

A man to his friend:

"Abe, why do you think there are so many justified divorces?"

"I guess that's because there are too many unjustified marriages..."

An extramarital affair is like a military operation. It involves three stages.

- Stage I: Conception
- Stage II: Execution
- Stage III: Termination

And, not unlike the launching of a military campaign, there are direct hits and collateral damage. The common denominator in an affair is a perennial sense of uneasiness, fear, and, on occasion, guilt.

Stage I: Conception Phase

The conception phase is the most benign for the cardiac patient. He or she selects a prospective candidate for the affair. Communication develops between them—but without any serious emotional compromise or significant physical contact. At this point, the affair looks like a teenager's game. There's temptation and fantasy, but that's about it.

The good thing about Stage I is that timely withdrawal prevents future complications.

Murphy's Law: If Something Can Go Wrong, It Will

A man to his friend, philosophically:
"Fred, why in the world do we make so many mistakes?"
"I guess that's because we plan them carefully!"
"Oh, man, is she gorgeous, sensuous, beautiful. What a woman!" That is the way Dick described his new extramarital conquest. He was a corporate executive, she was a secretary. They had already had a couple of amorous encounters at a Ramada Inn. One day, he arrived at the hotel with a couple of bottles of fine wine and some gastronomic delicacies. She wanted to ask him something, but didn't know how to do it. Finally, she overcame her shyness and made her request. She wanted to have sex while her hands were tied with rope to the bedposts. Her fantasy was to "to get raped" by her lover. "No sadomasochistic stuff, really. Just a little nothing, an innocent satisfaction of a long-repressed desire."

Dick was taken by surprise and wasn't sure how to respond, but he quickly adjusted and was willing to please her. He needed a rope.

Actually, he needed several pieces of rope, or strings, or whatever. All that mattered was to find something to please "the most adorable and sexiest creature you've ever seen in your life."

He ran down to the registration clerk and asked for directions to a shop where he could buy rope. He was told there was a fishing supplies store nearby, where he could get what he needed. He drove to the place as fast as he could. He bought the rope and a knife to cut the rope into pieces. The knife was so sharp, that "you could have used it to cut cement like a piece of salami."

He rushed back to the motel room and found his girlfriend stretching her beautiful anatomy all over the bed, half-naked, staring at him with a romantic look that radiated lust—and the effects of the half-bottle of wine she had already drained. He was so overwhelmed with emotion and excitement that his hands began to tremble. He tied one of her wrists to the bed. As he maneuvered to do the same with the other, he cut his finger and started to bleed profusely.

The wound was deep and the bleeding uncontrollable. The fact that he was taking an anticoagulant because of a heart condition made a bad situation worse. In a few seconds, there were spots of blood staining his pants, shirt, bed sheets, and more. He realized his best option was to exit the motel immediately and go to an emergency room. His girlfriend showed solidarity by following him with her own car. From his cellular phone, he called his wife to tell her that he had accidentally cut his finger and was now heading toward the hospital.

What he didn't count on was his wife's desire to assist him. She, too, went to the emergency room. There she saw her husband's hand being held and kissed by a woman with her clothes stained with blood. She immediately put it all together, said nothing, and left.

A couple of hours later, when Dick returned home, he was thrown out of the house in the presence of his two kids. What followed next was a devastating divorce, divorce attorneys, psychologists for the entire family, and serious financial losses. His increasing shortness of breath, palpitations, and chest pains reminded him that he was a cardiac patient, and that his cardiologist had strongly advised him to have "a stress-free life, as much as possible."

Stage II: Execution Phase

The execution phase introduces inconveniences. Life has changed. The affair takes off, and the couple is ready to meet at a hotel room. Hiding becomes official, and sunglasses are compulsory for both protagonists, even during night hours. In the parking lot or hotel lobby, they look more like CIA operatives working on a secret mission than lovers. When the hotel room door finally opens with a nervously handled key that never seems to work the first time, the glorious moment is near and the heart starts pounding. "Oh, man, this is exciting. This is the real life, not what I have at home. Oh, God, I shouldn't have said that. Come on, no guilt. This is the time for action, not guilt. Let's enjoy the moment. I'm getting a green light. What the hell am I waiting for?"

And sex occurs. Tensions are relaxed, at least for the moment—*and if* no freak accidents occur. (Remember Murphy's Law, and see "Risks of an Affair in a Hotel Room" on page 104).

Stage III: Termination Phase

It takes two people to start a relationship, and it takes the same number to end it, discreetly or otherwise. And the termination phase is not always an easy passage. One thing is certain, however; Stage III is the most disturbing of all the stages involved in an affair.

I've seen men and women who want to end an affair, but their lover does not. Whether this results from a "fatal attraction," or from a vicious attempt at revenge, extortion, or both, it probably doesn't matter. At some point, the mess becomes so sticky and disgusting that it is very difficult to come out of it unhurt. Unexpected developments may make a bad situation even worse: the woman gets pregnant, the man or the woman is infected with highly contagious genital herpes, and so on. The distress resulting from these situations is difficult to describe.

One of my male patients got involved with the wrong woman. He requested an urgent appointment with me, not so much because of his heart condition, but because he was so desperate that he wanted the opinion of a friend. He needed to find a viable way out of a desperate situation. He was trapped "in a huge spider web" with his mistress. When he decided he no longer wanted the relationship and broke the news to her, her face "turned green and purple," he said. She responded with anger:

"Finished, kaput? Is that what you're telling me? Who do you think you're talking to? Do I look like a bimbo? Is that what you think of me? When we began dating, you sounded so romantic. Every time I got undressed, your eyes rolled up and down. Now you look at me like a zombie. You mean to tell me that it's all over? Listen to me, bastard—don't you dare give up on me now. If you do, I promise—I'm gonna tell your wife, your children, your boss, your church, your friends, and your barber. Everybody will know what you did. There will be no peace for you. You're not going to have an easy ride. I can guarantee you that."

He ended the affair, and her retribution took place right on schedule. He lost everything he had—his home, his family and friends, his money. He resumed the heavy drinking that he had given up years before and went back to smoking. One year later, he underwent quadruple coronary bypass surgery.

PART THREE

COMMUNICATION WITH YOUR DOCTOR AND YOUR PARTNER

Chapter 10

How to Talk to Your Doctor

Silence is golden, as long as you talk later...

Conversations between you and your doctor serve more than one purpose. They can reveal abilities and shortcomings on both sides, and they can establish compatibility. They also help develop a rapport and confidence in the physician, or help you decide that you need another doctor or healthcare professional (HCP), whatever the case may be.

If you have reservations about expressing your thoughts about sex with your doctor, try a written introduction (See the Questionnaires below). You may be more comfortable doing that than having a direct, regular conversation with the professional. This can at least serve as a temporary solution until you and your doctor feel more adequate discussing intimacies in greater depth.

Always keep in mind that, regardless of your good intentions to initiate or expand a dialogue with your physician about sexual concerns, he or she may not be receptive or comfortable and might avoid the subject, or attempt channeling it in a different direction.

This kind of situation may also happen in reverse. The doctor may offer you an invitation to express your sexual questions, and for a number of different reasons (shyness, sense of privacy, or insufficient rapport with your doctor), you decide to evade the sexual issue, at least, for the moment.

Both of these questionnaires give you a general idea about the most common questions that you, as a cardiac patient, might want to ask to your doctor.

Questionnaire 1 includes questions you should ask your family doctor, internist, nurse practitioner, or cardiologist.

Questionnaire 2 lists a number of questions you should ask a psychologist, psychiatrist, or sex therapist.

THE APPROPRIATE TIME TO ASK QUESTIONS, AND THE USE OF THE SEXUAL PERFORMANCE QUESTIONNAIRES

Questions on sexual activity should be asked when recovery from a cardiac crisis is under way. If you have unstable cardiac symptoms, insufficient information about the status of your heart, or a poor convalescence, you should postpone the questions.

It is important to keep in mind that questions posed to the doctor by the patient should be limited to the technical aspects of sexual activity in relation to the patient's specific heart condition. Additional interrogation involving psychological, emotional, or relationship conflicts, as well as a number of detailed sexual interaction issues of a very intimate and private nature, are not applicable.

Let me give you a few examples of how, as a cardiologist, I pose some questions to the patient and the way I do it.

I may advise the use of the "on top" position to a man or a woman because he or she needs to place the thorax vertically to reduce or avoid chest congestion. This tends to happen when the heart muscle is weak. The suggestion is appropriate. But I will not ask the patient if he or she enjoys that position. That question is intrusive.

Another situation:

I may find it advisable for the patient (a man or a woman) to try oral-genital sex if I feel that at a particular time the maneuver would be less taxing for him/her than vaginal intercourse and if the patient accepts being counseled on this issue, but I'd never ask the patient if he/she ever had oral-genital contact previously.

The physician needs to understand the boundaries, the limits that must be drawn when the patient is questioned about sex. The professional should answer the questions that pertain to the patient's sexual activity in relation to the patient's heart disease.

Other issues—that are of great importance, to be sure—such as conflicts of the marital relationship, lack of orgasms, complaints related to the inadequacy of sexual stimulation by the partner, influence on a present sexual dysfunction due to past sexual abuse, sexual boredom, and a host of other psychological or relational problems, should be gently deferred to the psychotherapist or sex therapist.

THE CONFIDENTIALITY ISSUE

Different HCP do different things. Medical records are an important aspect of medical practice, but when it comes to sexual issues, I do not register details. I might mention in a consultation report dictated for a consulting physician that the patient suffers from a sexual dysfunction and erectile failure, or that a female patient has vaginal pain during intercourse. Beyond that, what the patient or the patient's sexual partner shares in strict confidence will be buried with me.

Usually, there's no need to record the patient's intimate confessions. At times, a very close rapport is established between patient and professional and sensitive things are said.

If I have a need to record a delicate and compromising confession for future reference, I use what I call my "X-files." These notes are kept in a secret place at my office and contain no names. To assure total confidentiality and secrecy they are labeled by letters and numbers such as DLTX 20091. This identification is only known by the patient. If he or she never shows me that number, the chart will never be identified. Not even by myself.

SEXUAL PERFORMANCE QUESTIONNAIRE 1

These questions apply to patients recovering from acute cardiac events, such as a myocardial infarction, balloon angioplasty and stent implantation, heart valve repair or replacement, coronary bypass surgery, pacemaker or intracardiac defibrillator implantation, cardiomyopathy, significant arrhythmias, unstable angina, syncope (black-out spell), congestive heart failure, hypertension, and thoracic and abdominal aneurysms.

The same questions also apply to all forms of chronic heart disease.

1. When can I resume sexual activity?
2. What methods or sexual positions should I use?
3. Is there any position I should avoid, or be particularly careful with?
4. Should I avoid vaginal penetration for some time because it is too strenuous? (Applies to both sexes).
5. What should I do if I develop chest pains or shortness of breath during intercourse?
6. When should I call the doctor or 911?
7. Should I use nitroglycerin tablets or other cardiac medications prior to, during, or following intercourse?
8. Can I take several drugs at the same time? If so, what side effects could I have? Example: Sometimes diuretics can cause hypotension (abnormally low blood pressure), and so

do other drugs, such as beta-blockers, calcium blockers, and others. If a sublingual nitroglycerin is taken, the blood pressure may become even lower and cause dizziness or fainting.

9. Which of the medications that I take could affect my sexual function?

10 What instructions should my sexual partner have?

11. May I ask you questions personally about my sexual performance, or would you prefer I consult another professional?

12. I'd like to consult a psychologist, psychiatrist, or sex therapist. Can you recommend someone?

13. I have one or more of the following problems:
    - Decreased sexual desire
    - Genital pain prior to intercourse
    - No erections
    - Painful ejaculation
    - Painful erections
    - Premature ejaculation
    - Soft erections
    - Trouble reaching orgasm
    - Vaginal pain during intercourse
    - Other difficulties

14. What should I do next?

15. Can I take Viagra, Levitra, or Cialis?

16. Can you describe to me the available treatment options that deal with my sexual dysfunction?

17. My wife had a heart attack one year ago and she's multiorgasmic. She's very intense during intimacy. I'm afraid that something could happen to her while making love. How dangerous that can be for her condition?

18. I'd like you to be my doctor, but I prefer to discuss sex with another professional. Can you help me with a recommendation?

SEXUAL PERFORMANCE QUESTIONNAIRE 2

The following are some of the questions that should be asked to a psychotherapist or sex therapist.

1. I had conflicts related to intimacy with previous sexual partners. How much is this background is affecting my present sexual dysfunction?
2. My sexual partner and I do not interact well sexually.
3. My spouse and I keep mutual resentments and the tension is felt all the time.
4. My mate is imposing restrictions on my sexual play.
5. My partner is not sensitive to my needs.
6. Our sexual styles are very different.
7. Our preferences about the time to have sex are very different.
8. I am oversexed and my [husband] is undersexed.
9. I was sexually abused as a child and also during adulthood.
10. My sexual difficulties actually preceded my heart condition.
11. I use my heart disease as an excuse to avoid sex with my spouse.
12. I'd like to change many things during intimacy. I'm getting bored.
13. I'd like to have sex 5 times a week and my partner wants it once every 2 weeks.
14. My mate does not appear to enjoy intimacy with me.
15. My spouse is very sexually demanding. Sometimes, I feel I just can't take it any longer!

16. My sexual dysfunction started suddenly (or gradually).
    What does that mean?

17. Is masturbation allowed? And what about masturbating the
    sexual partner?

18. There are sexual positions I enjoy but my partner dislikes.
    Is there a way of finding a solution to this problem?

19. My mate gets sexually aroused fairly quickly but I don't.
    Can you explain to me why?

There are more questions about sexuality cardiac patients may have
for the primary care physician, nurse practitioner, or cardiologist of the
type seen in the first questionnaire, and for the psychotherapist or sex
therapist in the second. I have just mentioned the most common.

How adequately the professional will respond to your questions,
you'll never know until you ask them. The questionnaires will help you
identify concerns and difficulties in sexual functioning of yourself and
your partner and facilitate the communication with the professional in a
more organized and effective manner. It will also contribute to a better
understanding of the couple's difficulties and that is, of course, absolutely essential for their eventual resolution.

PROBLEMS WHEN DISCUSSING SEX WITH YOUR DOCTOR

It would be arrogant and untruthful to state that physicians do everything
right. No one can make that claim. The inescapable reality is that human
beings are not perfect, even if they happen to be doctors. Becoming
aware of one's mistakes means dealing with wounded pride. What can be
done about the mistakes we've made? Only one thing, I believe: doing
whatever is necessary to avoid repeating them. Humor, humility, and
humanity are invaluable in making the criticism more palatable.

While this book is primarily written for the cardiac patient, I hope that healthcare professionals and undergraduates will also derive some benefit from it.

In the following pages, you'll notice that my recommendations for errors committed by professionals are addressed to them.

As far as *you* are concerned, the usefulness of these observations is that you'll become familiar with some professional imperfections that, properly recognized, will prevent or minimize the discomforts and inconveniences these might cause.

Doctors fail to communicate with patients on sexual issues for a number of reasons. I know what those reasons are, partly because I lived through most of them at one point or another in the course of my career. So, do not think for a moment that during the practice of my profession for many years, I was the kind of physician who never made mistakes. I've surely made them. Because I respect my profession and the medical practitioners who commit themselves to do the best possible job in dealing with their patients, I do believe that attempts to achieve excellence in the practice of medicine should begin by the admission and recognition of our own imperfections, and also do whatever we can to correct them.

With that constructive and positive idea in mind, let me share them with you.

Lack of Familiarity with the Subject

PATIENT: "Would you answer some questions about sex?"

PHYSICIAN: "Why should I? I'm just a doctor!"

Most medical schools don't place enough emphasis on teaching sexual counseling, and what the students do learn does not translate into effective action. The same applies to post-graduate training programs (intern-ships and residencies). The study of medical conditions with a sexual com-ponent, such as AIDS, gonorrhea, and the like, is amply examined, but per-sonal aspects of a patient's sexuality receive considerably less attention.

Recommended solution: Sexual counseling for the cardiac patient should be part of the educational curriculum at medical schools through lectures, courses, and workshops. Doctors also need more training about interviewing and counseling couples together.

Academic Numbness
PATIENT: "Doctor, I had a heart attack six weeks ago, and you have not advised me on what to do about sex. Can you tell me why?"

PHYSICIAN: "Would you believe it? I couldn't find enough information on this in the best cardiology textbooks!"

Some of the most prestigious cardiology publications in the United States—ones whose collaborators are distinguished professors, clinicians, and researchers—fail to offer any substantial discussion of the problems that relate to sex and the cardiac patient. The subject is barely men-tioned. Why? I don't know. To me, it remains an unresolved mystery.

Recommended solution: There should be a radical departure from the current practice of ignoring the subject of sex and heart disease. Future publications should address the issue in a comprehensive manner.

Too Little Time Available
PATIENT: "Doctor, why is it that you spend so little time with your patients?"

PHYSICIAN: "I guess I'm too busy practicing medicine!"

Hard work and commitment are essential components of human progress, but there are limits. Exceeding those limits is asking for trouble.

Doctors often need to do things fast. Fast and well. But speed narrows the margin of safety. In particular, a certain amount of time is needed for fruitful patient/doctor interaction. If the dialogue is rushed, the professional appears insensitive, inattentive, or incompetent. Patients may forgive occasional abruptness, but repetitive behavior of this kind generates distrust and disappointment.

One day, years ago, while working in Miami Beach, I had so many hospitalized patients that in order to see them all, I decided to get up at 4:30 A.M. I realized the timing was terrible, since the patients would be asleep, but I saw no viable alternative: To do my job right, I had to get up that early.

That day, I entered a semiprivate hospital room, turned on the lights, touched the shoulder of my elderly patient, and said:

"Good morning, Sam. Please wake up."

"What the hell are you doing in the hospital at this hour?"

"I'm making rounds, Sam. I have a lot of work to do."

"What?

"I HAVE A LOT OF WORK TO DO!"

"Shhh, you're waking everybody up. Where's my hearing aid?"

"Here it is, Sam. I just gave you your glasses and your hearing aid. In case you also want your dentures, they're sitting on the table. Sam, don't you understand? I'm in a hurry. Please, tell me: Do you have any complaints today?"

"Yes, I have Blue Cross, Blue Shield, and Medicare."

"Sam, you still don't hear a damn thing. I think I'd better see you tomorrow?

"Tomorrow? You haven't seen me today yet!"

"Sam, I've got to go."

"Okay, Okay, go, but don't work so hard. You must eat on time, have a good rest. And take weekends off, and vacations. I always see you running. That's not good!

"Thanks for the advice, Sam."

"Listen, I'm not a doctor, but I know how to take care of myself. Otherwise, I'd never have reached 85. I hope you'll live that long!"

"Thanks again, Sam. You're a sweet man!"

And those were the days, my friend.

Recommended solution: Excessive work may impair judgment or cause errors of omission, both of which are detrimental to the patient and the doctor.

Excessive Fatigue

PATIENT: "Doctor, you look very sleepy. Would you like to see me at another time?"

PHYSICIAN: "NO! Not even in my wildest dreams!"

The physical energy that many doctors display is remarkable. In fact, their energy may seem inexhaustible, but it is not. When fatigue sets in, it's easier to make a mistake or miscalculation. This is dangerous not only to patients but also to doctors. Physicians have lost their lives in car accidents following long hours of intensive hospital work.

Or consider this scenario: The doctor is extremely tired and falls asleep while interviewing a patient, just for an instant, the same way exhausted people lose control for a few seconds while driving on the expressway. I presume this is an extremely rare occurrence.

A female patient who had trusted a doctor for many years described such an incident to me. While she was consulting him about intimate problems she was having with her husband, the very tired physician began dozing off. Suddenly, he snapped out of his brief somnolent interlude and made an extraordinary effort to remain awake. Not surprisingly, she decided to change doctors. As she related the story to me, she made this comment, with a cute touch of humor: "This was a no win situation for me: Every time I wanted to talk to my husband about orgasms, he fell asleep. When I was ready to consult a professional about guidance for my problem, he did the same thing. I said to myself, 'What is this? Am I running out of luck? Am I that boring?'"

Recommended solution to exhausted doctors: Find a replacement for a few hours and get some rest. Then, take a cold shower and drink two gallons of undiluted Cuban coffee. Look at your face in the mirror. If you conclude it's yours and no one else's, brush your teeth, gargle for 2 minutes, practice a re-entry smile, and dutifully go back to work.

Inappropriate Character and Personality

PATIENT: "Doctor, can you help me to overcome my sexual inhibitions?"

PHYSICIAN: "Of course, but I've yet to get rid of my own!"

Some physicians feel uneasy talking about sex and react with noticeable swallowing of saliva. When the patient asks an unexpected question, the doctor's gulping becomes a reflex, and the interviewer follows suit.

Simultaneous gulping by patient and professional is indicative of a momentous landmark in their communication. It strongly suggests that both are made of the same fabric and will either enjoy total and unconditional understanding, or they'll never be willing to see each other again.

Recommended solution: More exposure and training in sexology, psychology, and communications skills at medical school and during postgraduate training.

Attitude

A PHYSICIAN TO A COLLEAGUE: "John, do you ever talk to your patients about sex?"

COLLEAGUE: "Of course, I do—if I'm left with no other choice!"

Some physicians simply dislike talking about sex, just as they dislike talking about orthopedics or dermatology. As a result, they cut short any conversation that relates to sex.

Recommended solution: The physician should provide the patient with written educational material.

Interruptions during Patient Interviews

Interruptions are highly disruptive and should be avoided as much as possible. For example, the patient is talking to the doctor and the phone rings every few minutes, the nurse or the secretary makes frequent appearances to ask questions, or the physician walks out of the room more often than he or she should.

Recommended solution: Have the office manager educate personnel about avoiding interruptions unless there's an emergency.

Mistaken Assumptions by the Physician

Assumptions are a poor substitute for knowledge.

Looks can be misleading. When you see a bodybuilder on the front page of a magazine, you may be tempted to think that he is a sexual superman. In real life, despite all his beautiful muscles, that man may be totally impotent. Gorgeous women who talk about sex, dress sexy, and convey erotic hopes to those attracted to them may sometimes be the most frigid and sexually unresponsive women during intimacy.

On the other hand, sick people, who may look physically unattractive and have serious physical disabilities, may be the most sensuous, passionate, and skillful lovers. When it comes to guessing about people's sexual abilities, therefore, forget about it: I don't know; you don't know; nobody knows, except their partners.

Let me give you several examples where I badly underestimated a patient's potential to engage in lovemaking.

These examples teach us to be cautious about estimating the sexual potential of patients who suffer serious disabilities. In all of the above situations, I never suspected that these individuals were able or willing to do what they did. It seems, however, that for some people, sex may be the last bulb that goes off.

Recommended solution: Never judge a person's sexuality based upon his or her appearance. If there's a Pandora's box in our souls, this is it.

Bad Timing

Patients should never be pressed to talk about sex. They should just be given the opportunity.

A doctor who talks about sex with a patient who is not in a receptive mood may regret it. If the patient views sex as a challenge that he or she cannot meet, the reaction may be one of frustration and anger.

Years ago, while making teaching rounds with interns and residents at the University Hospital, I stressed the importance of talking to patients about sexual concerns. A young graduate felt compelled to apply these concepts quickly. He chose one of his ward patients, a man in his forties, who had been a war veteran. He suffered from chronic

Stories: How Old Is Too Old?

A 76-year-old woman had advanced emphysema and required oxygen around the clock. She had to be transported by wheelchair because her marked fatigue prohibited her from walking. She enjoyed sex regularly with a much younger lover and stated she had never been so happy.

Her three daughters resented her relationship and thought that at her age, and in poor health, she had to be out of her mind to do something like that. The patient disagreed and kept her lover and her smile.

A man in his mid-sixties, suffering from severe lung and heart disease, disabled because of chronic fatigue and shortness of breath, required two hospitalizations in a 2-month period for critical recurrences of his condition. I suspected these life-threatening episodes were related to sexual activity because in both admissions to the hospital, the routine urinalysis reported "large quantity of spermatozoids." His wife confirmed my suspicions and stated that her husband "demanded regular sex twice a week. When he was healthy, and for a period of many years, he used to have sex two to three times a day." When I warned him against sexual activity after surviving a cardiac arrest, his response was one of uncontrolled laughter.

A 64-year-old woman suffered from baldness, severe rheumatoid arthritis, heart disease, recurrent gastrointestinal bleeding, and chronic anemia. She was a picture of devastation. However, her husband was very concerned because she was "oversexed and multi-orgasmic." He was afraid that her passionate lovemaking "could one day stop her heart."

depression, severe anxiety, panic attacks, occasional uncontrollable violent behavior, and advanced physical and mental disability. In addition, he had a very limited income, two dysfunctional children, and an unhappy marital relationship. The well-motivated doctor brought up the subject of sex for possible counseling. The reaction was swift. The patient became upset and said: "I can't believe you're talking to me about sex when I can barely stand on my feet! Leave it to someone else, will you? I have so many other things to worry about."

The physician was dismayed and embarrassed. He told me: "I think it'll be a very long time before I ask anybody any questions about sex." I went with the trainees to a room where we could all relax with a cup of coffee, and I shared with the young physicians my points of view on the general way I try to establish a conversation with a patient about intimate situations:

- ❤ "Develop the ability to communicate. Sex is a very sensitive subject, and an acceptable level of communication is not possible with every patient. For various reasons, some patients don't want to bother with this theme and refuse to talk about it with the physician, sexual partner, and even themselves.

- ❤ "Always keep in mind your knowledge limitations about psychology and sexuality unless you were formally trained in these subjects. Some patients, who find you a compassionate and attentive listener, may inadvertently try to convert you into a psychotherapist. Don't forget for a moment that you are not one.

- ❤ "The main role of the primary-care physician or cardiologist is to disclose the existence of a conflict and to provide guidance. Psychotherapy is a complex subject, and it is the domain of the psychotherapist. If the solution to a problem is obvious, simple, and straightforward, the patient can be advised immediately. If the solution isn't clear, recommend a professional you trust.

- ❤ "Conversations with clients about sexual issues should never be rushed. If you have a busy schedule, let the patient know, and reschedule the interview.

♥ "The physician's personal taste and views on sexuality and morality are irrelevant and non-applicable. In the practice of medicine, the only thing that matters is the patient's problems, never the doctor's problems. By being the recipient of intimate confessions, the professional is granted a vote of confidence and a special privilege. This merits reciprocation and a conscientious effort to apply your knowledge as honestly and as wisely as you can."

Some of the observations I made in this chapter are potentially more easily correctable than others. Quite often, even a modestly-improved performance by the professional, in association with a higher level of awareness and a sense of compassion for a patient's dilemma is sufficient to make an important contribution to his or her state of physical, mental, and sexual health.

WHAT IS A PATIENT SUPPOSED TO DO WHEN HIS OR HER HEALTH CARE PRACTITIONER SHOWS ANY OF THE DEFICIENCIES LISTED IN THIS CHAPTER?

I've just described inadequate responses by healthcare professionals when dealing with sex and heart disease. Recommended solutions were offered to medical practitioners because I referred to their faults and omissions.

From your own perspective as a patient, you've got to decide what to do when you face such situations. Do you want to continue under the care of your current doctor, or not?

DO NOT ACT IMPULSIVELY

The relationship between a patient and a doctor does not have to be perfect, although it should definitely be a good one. The selection of a physician implies that in certain instances, your life may depend upon her/his actions. That alone justifies the need to be under the care of a competent professional.

Now, are competent practitioners only those who discuss sexual issues with their patients?

The answer is: NO!

I know excellent physicians who do not like to talk about sex with their patients. They are quite prudish by reason of education, tradition, religion, or family values. Some will barely touch the surface of the sexual issue that must be dealt with, but will quickly withdraw.

In such cases, the first questionnaire may help you and your doctor communicate.

If you have a good doctor who evades sex talk but is otherwise a good doctor, in every sense of the word, keep her/him. Read this book, learn as much as you can, and then present the questions that concern you. Limit those to the most important ones.

I said something at the beginning of this chapter that I'm going to repeat at the end of it. In my own practice of medicine, I was guilty of the errors and omissions I described here. Motivation and dedication hopefully made me a better doctor. That is exactly what I suggest to those professionals who need to improve their performance on the subject of sex and the cardiac patient.

Always respect the professional who is honest and capable. Sex talk is important, but other fundamental aspects of the professional's character take precedence: the doctor's personality, qualifications, efficiency, reliability, humanity, and decency ought to be considered a priority and far less negotiable than sex talk, as important as it is.

Chapter 11

Your Sexual Partner: Communication is Key

WIFE: "Tony, why do you speak to me so softly?"

HUSBAND: "I guess I'm afraid you'll hear what I'm trying to tell you!"

Stress results from our perception of events. The brain decides what is stressful and what is not. When the brain makes up its mind and defines a situation as stressful, it channels the psychological/physical reactions into a constructive or destructive path. The former path converts stress into positive forces that can be challenging and stimulating. The latter path translates stress into a force that is disruptive and harmful. Typically, you see this kind of stress in an unhappy marriage or other committed relationship. It is like a toxic breeze that permeates the pores of your skin, affects every cell of your body, and aborts every attempt to achieve happiness and contentment.

Unless you find a solution to your unhappiness—and thus a way to alleviate the stress—one day you'll notice that your shoes are too tight, that a beautiful sunny day isn't any different from a rainy one, that the heartburn caused by the best homemade tomato sauce feels like an inextinguishable fire, and that getting into bed with your mate is a nightmare even before you start dreaming.

Marital discord can get ugly indeed. Turbulent relationships are, among other things, a disappointment. You never imagined that the person you loved so much would one day turn into a symbol of unrepressed confrontation. Fortunately, the situation need not be permanent. Problems at home can often be worked out. Disagreements can exist, but without being expressed destructively. Divergent opinions can be exposed at the negotiating table, and, although viewpoints may differ, life continues without noxious regressions.

Love is the best hope for relationship conflicts, because loving is forgiving and unconditional acceptance. It is the great neutralizer. Love is a mysterious force, and mysteries, by definition, don't have a reasonable explanation. That's why many people fall in love and later try to figure out how it happened. In a way, this "incomprehensibility" is what makes love work. That's the beauty of love: It obviates the need to understand the other person.

The loss of love, however, is the beginning of the end. A pattern of emotional indifference follows. Given enough time, partners lose respect for each other. I'm not referring to a few words expressed in anger, but the real thing—the authentic loss of feeling and sensitivity toward the mate.

From that point on the couple will have to make a choice: confrontation at home versus ablation at court. In other words, it's going to be a household fighting like cats and dogs forever (which is not good), or getting a divorce (which is not cheap). Actually, there is a third alternative—passionless toleration.

During a cardiac crisis, the status of the marital relationship is particularly important. The recovery period is a vulnerable one. The patient is physically debilitated and emotionally drained. A battered heart can only take so much anguish. And since the heart doesn't always warn us in advance when it calls it quits, we should treat it with respect.

WHEN YOU NEED HELP: WHO SHOULD YOU CONSULT?

Marital relationship conflicts involve numerous variants. It is essential to identify as clearly as possible what these are and what role and impact each one of them has in the dynamics of the relationship.

The reason for this is that every reason for disagreement, resentment, or antagonism requires individual attention. If the presence of an unwanted relative living at home is the cause of the sexual dysfunction, or this results from aggravation and discord from the gestures of an intrusive family, one must primarily focus on those issues and try to find a solution for those problems, rather than placing all the emphasis on the sexual dysfunction.

In such cases, a family counselor is preferable to a sex therapist.

If one of the sexual partners suffers from a bipolar disorder, schizophrenia, or a severe personality disorder, and the couple experiences sexual friction, a psychiatrist should be consulted.

Persons who were brought up in a dysfunctional home environment and have difficulties to relating to other people, at the work place, or have personality disorders that derail relationships and are unable to be sexually happy or make their partners happy, might benefit best from a consultation with a psychologist.

Those who have sexual inhibitions, or do not know exactly how to please the sexual partner with reasonable requests because of unfounded fears or prejudices, find intimacy boring, or want to be taught specific positions and techniques to enjoy sex to the best of their capacities will benefit from a few sessions with a sex therapist.

Often, a couple has several problems at the same time. It's better to separate them and proceed with their analysis one by one.

THE ART OF COMMUNICATION

WIFE: "John, c'est que tu parlay Francais?"

HUSBAND: "Sorry, Maria, I don't speak Italian!"

The months that follow a heart attack, cardiac surgery, or a temporarily disabling heart condition test the strength of a relationship and its potential for growth. This recovery period provides an opportunity to share and show empathy, solidarity, and companionship. When flexibility and patience prevail, the rewards can be immense.

For those who need to improve their relationship or who cannot resolve their differences, I suggest reading *Making It as a Couple,* by Dr. Allen Fay. This book is about relationship problems and their possible solutions. See Chapter 12 for a conversation I had with him and one of the most influential psychologists of modern times, Dr. Arnold A. Lazarus.

Dr. Fay starts by saying, "The fact is that most relationships don't work. Either they don't work at all, they don't work for too long, or they don't work very well." Why? The simplest answer is that "most couples don't know how to make them work." Dr. Fay claims that "we go through life without the necessary skills for creating and maintaining relationships."

I don't disagree with these notions at all, although I'd like to add a personal note: It's my belief that when you have the right "chemistry" in a relationship, you don't need to exhaust all your energy to make it successful. In contrast, when you select the wrong partner, the best therapist in the world may find it impossible to reassemble the pieces of a badly fractured marriage.

In relationships, as in many aspects of life, there's a point of no return. This means that you should try to solve problems while there still remains some degree of flexibility and goodwill on both sides.

137

Dr. Fay reminds us that, when confronting a failing relationship, you have four alternatives:

- Accept it for what it is.
- Suffer and resent it.
- End the relationship.
- Work at making it better.

His book deals with the fourth alternative. He describes 54 relationship "traps," and provides specific remedies for dealing with every one of them. Among the traps Dr. Fay features are:

- Appealing to or quoting third parties for support
- Being inattentive
- Being right
- Blaming
- Confusing the person with the deed
- Criticizing
- Devaluing partner's contributions or accomplishments
- Disapproving
- Displaying negative dramatic behavior
- Doing a good deed sourly
- Failing to respond positively
- Giving orders
- Interrogating your partner
- Invalidating partner's perceptions
- Jealousy
- Making accusations
- Making negative comparisons
- Punishing the positive
- Reciting past grievances

- Regretting
- Saying no
- Self-justifying
- Taking credit
- Threatening
- Universalizing your own opinion
- Using "always" or "never"
- Using a double standard
- Using psychological warfare

...and the list goes on.

If you choose to work at improving your relationship, you have to invest time and effort. You also need:

- Awareness
- Motivation
- Mechanisms (methods or techniques to improve the relationship)

Due to denial or insufficient analysis, it's possible that you don't fully understand your marital conflicts. Stress may disconnect you from reality and blur the whole picture. Allen Fay's book will help you get out of the shadows and move your life in the right direction.

HEART DISEASE, SEX, AND A FAILED MARITAL RELATIONSHIP

A professional who listens only to one party will never accurately know what's going on in a relationship.

Bob and Mary had been my patients for many years. They were in their mid-sixties and had been married for a long time. Friction between them was constant. You could see daggers coming from their eyes, and they both exuded resentment. I saw them at my office following his recent acute myocardial infarction.

Dr. Chapunoff (Dr. C.): "Bob, I've given you instructions about everything related to your condition. Well, almost everything, since we haven't discussed sex yet. Since Mary is here, I'd like to ask you if I can help you in any way."

Bob: "I don't know."

Mary: "What do you mean, you 'don't know?' What are your plans? To avoid sex forever?"

Bob: "I didn't say that."

Mary: "You didn't say that, but that's what you meant!"

Bob: "Oh, come on. Don't start fighting. I just had a heart attack. I'm trying to recover, and here you come, bothering me again. Give me a break, will you?"

Mary: "I want you to recover, and after you get well, I want you to pay attention to me for a change."

Bob: "I will, I will."

Mary: "You've been telling me you 'will' for the past 35 years. How much longer am I supposed to wait? I'm not getting any younger. Don't you see that?"

Bob: "Of course, I do."

Mary: "Yeah, right."

Bob: "Dr. Chapunoff, I'm beginning to sweat. She really pisses me off. I think I'm having an angina attack. Where the hell did I put my nitroglycerin tablets?" (He searches nervously in his pockets).

Mary: "Here they are." (She takes a nitroglycerin tablet from her purse). "If it wasn't for me, you'd be dead already."

Bob: "Yeah, and I'd be better off."

Mary: "You never appreciate anything I do for you. I've been helping you for almost half a century, and this is the way you pay me back."

Bob: "Sure, sure, you saved my life and gave me three heart attacks."

Dr. C: "Hold it, right there, both of you. Now, it's my turn. Please, from now on, until we complete this interview, let me have control of this conversation. If I let you say what you want, you'll never stop hurting and insulting each other. You've given me a headache, and I think I'm having palpitations from watching both of you carrying on like this."

Mary: "Oh, Dr. Chapunoff, I'm so sorry. I feel terrible. We shouldn't give you this aggravation. Are you okay? Here, try this, put a nitroglycerin tablet under your tongue."

Dr. C: "No, thank you, Mary. I don't need it—at least, not yet. All I'm trying to do is to have a rational conversation. Do you understand?"

Mary: "Yes, at least, I do."

Bob: "That's right, she's the smart one. I'm the moron. I understand nothing."

Dr. C: "Let me ask you, is this the way you 'normally' communicate your thoughts?"

Bob: "Sometimes it's much worse."

Mary: "We've been doing this for so long, I think we've gotten used to it."

Bob: "That's ridiculous."

Mary: "Dr. Chapunoff, if you have a few more minutes, I'll tell you what it is. If nothing else, I'm going to feel relieved."

Dr. C: "Please, Mary, go ahead."

Mary: "My husband has always felt that sex is dirty. He doesn't like sex. He never did. When he was young, he told me he didn't want to have much sex because he was afraid of having more children. I was stupid enough those days to believe in such nonsense. Now that he's older and has a heart condition, he's found the perfect excuse. But my tolerance is gone. I tried everything—porno magazines, XXX-rated movies, and sexy underwear—anything that could stimulate him. What did I get? A lump of ice. Look at this..." She took four pornographic magazines out of her purse and threw them on my desk. "As a man, and tell me the truth, wouldn't you get excited with something like this?" She went on:

Mary: "What is he made of? Tell me. Why doesn't he become excited by things that all men get so excited about?"

Bob: "That's smut."

Mary: "Do you see? That's his typical reaction. I've told him many times, and I'm going to say it again: If he doesn't want to have sex with me, I'm going to find someone else. Don't say I didn't warn you." (She starts crying.)

Dr. C: "Listen Mary, and you too, Bob. When we started this conversation, my intention was to help you resume your sexual activity. I wasn't aware of your problems in that area. Obviously, you can't resume something you weren't doing before. The second point I want to make is that no cardiologist is capable of dealing with a situation like this. Your conflicts are long-standing and deep-rooted. You need to consult an expert in marital warfare."

Bob: "I'm not going to bother with that."

Dr. C: "This much is clear to me: Either you'll find a solution through counseling, or you'll continue feeling miserable for the rest of your lives. It's that simple."

Bob: "Eduardo, thank you for listening to all this crap."

Mary: "Yes, Ed, I thank you too."

Dr. C: "Good luck to both of you. Keep in touch."

Learning from your own and other people's experience, reading books on the subject, or consulting a specialist, can help your relationship problems. Whatever you decide, be aware of the conflicts before they cause serious damage to your relationship, your heart, or both. Solutions will have a better chance of success if they are implemented before your heart is at serious risk and you become psychologically and emotionally impaired. Don't let the wounds become too deep and tortuous. By the time they get to that state, it's very difficult to heal them.

CONCLUSION

Now, a few thoughts about the role of the primary-care physician and the cardiologist concerning the effect of the patient's personal problems on his or her mental and physical health.

Physicians are not experts in psychiatry or psychology. They should know their limitations, and at the same time be attuned to the emotional suffering of their patients.

Every professional's approach toward patients is different. A person who sees a cardiologist for preoperative clearance for gallbladder surgery, and who is probably never going to be examined again, does not have the rapport with this physician that is necessary for sharing many intimate details of his or her life. Several interviews may be needed to create the right atmosphere to tackle these delicate issues. It must be remembered that emotional/psychological disturbances can cause symptoms such as chest pain, shortness of breath, palpitations, and dizziness, among others. These may be indicative of either heart disease, or severe anxiety and stress.

Over the years, I've seen patients who did not respond to a variety of treatments for high blood pressure, chest pains, or pounding of the heart. The solution for their cardiac abnormalities or discomforts was not providing them with more pills, but understanding the stress-induced nature of their complaints. Whether the stress was related to domestic violence, a seriously dysfunctional relationship, or other reasons, the treatment approach, to be successful, required identification of the culprit.

Many people in our culture still rightly feel that being a doctor implies more than prescribing antibiotics or digitalis. They expect a degree of sensitivity that goes beyond the formalities of the case. We are not talking about interfering in anybody's private affairs, or providing psychiatric or psychological counseling that should be reserved for professionals versed in that field. We are talking about knowing what kind of problem the patient has, and what kind of counseling he or she needs.

Advances in medical technology, time constraints, and the myriad socioeconomic factors that currently affect the practice of medicine, should not lead us to forget that, in the midst of oxygen tanks, catheters, balloon angioplasties, and other surgical procedures, there are souls looking for solace and comfort. Physicians have a significant role in satisfying these needs in the now technical domain of medical practice.

Chapter 12

A Conversation with Two Experts in the Field of Human Interaction

Wisdom is the ultimate goal of knowledge.

Working on this book gave me a great deal of joy. I'd come home from my office in the evening, relax for a while, and then go to the word processor to do my writing. It became a routine—a nice, pleasant routine. But one day was special. It was the day that Drs. Arnold Lazarus and Allen Fay accepted my invitation to participate in this project by answering some questions I had for them. They are exceptionally talented psychotherapists who have had considerable influence on the field, on patients, and on students over several decades.

What you are going to read in this chapter are the questions I asked myself so many times during several decades of cardiology practice. You'll see that the questions go beyond the routine administration of medical care and drugs that I commonly give my patients.

I've always been under the impression that the majority of patients suffering from cardiovascular disease have created their own problems. Cardiovascular risk factors that contribute to myocardial infarctions and strokes—such as hypertension, obesity, high blood cholesterol levels, smoking, stress, and many others—wouldn't exist or would be far milder if psychological factors weren't involved. But they are—and very prominently and dangerously so.

Our emotional load, behavior, and interaction with other people are vital issues; when things go the wrong way, we have to face the consequences of our poor choices, our mistaken perceptions, and our improper decisions, all of which most of us have experienced at one time or another. And these could be prevented or minimized…if we only knew how.

If we then go back to the basics and search for the origin of sexual dysfunctions associated with heart disease, the central theme is also often psychological or relationship dysfunction. I've been repeatedly impressed by the frequency and pervasiveness of people's emotional and situational conflicts, and their disruptive power. And I've been as impacted by people's seeming inability to deal with them effectively.

Throughout the course of our lives, we learn from our own experiences or from those of others. Observation of other people's behavior and what results from their actions provides major learning opportunities. So, too, does reading instructive literature or consulting a psychotherapist. Most of us don't and can't learn enough from our own experiences. The problem with learning only from our own mistakes is that by the time we assimilate enough knowledge to conduct our lives in a reasonably effective manner, we have often paid an excessive price.

Unquestionably, there is something wrong with our preparedness to deal with complex and sometimes even simple life situations. Deficiencies are obvious at all levels.

- ❤ We neglect to take preventive and/or therapeutic measures against major health risks such as obesity, stress, and smoking, among others.

- We attempt to deal with critical conflicts and issues—financial hardship, job difficulties, relationship problems—without the special education and training essential to solving them.
- We don't take the necessary time, energy, and commitment required to repair the damage done to our physical and mental health. Consequently, some psychological wounds take longer to heal than necessary, while others cause permanent damage.

It is abundantly clear that we have to learn more about preventive interventions and human relations to avoid being pulverized when adversity puts us to the test. I also believe that we have to enlist the aid of those who can teach us what to do, when to do it, and how to do it. We need their knowledge, their analytical acumen, and their counseling. Then we need to learn how to apply that knowledge expediently and practically.

That's precisely the area in which psychotherapists Arnold Lazarus and Allen Fay excel. They focus on a "here and now" problem-solving approach. Their methods address the immediate conflict and stress the importance of behavioral change. They use techniques that are simple, accessible, direct, quick, and frequently successful.

It is impossible to separate your relationship with your partner and the conflicts and stress that come with that relationship, from sex, and that is why I've included this conversation with two renowned psychotherapists.

Before getting to the questions and answers, let me briefly describe our consultants' backgrounds.

Arnold A. Lazarus, Ph.D., is the Distinguished Professor Emeritus of Psychology at Rutgers University, a Diplomate of the American Board of Professional Psychology, and President of the Center for Multimodal

Psychological Services in Princeton, New Jersey. He has also served on the faculties of Stanford University, Temple University Medical School, and Yale University. He is a Fellow of the Academy of Clinical Psychology, and has received many honors and awards for his contributions to clinical theory and therapy, including two lifetime achievement awards and the prestigious Cummings *Psyche* award for his contributions to the field of behavioral health.

His multimodal therapy approach is one of the first, if not the most enduring, integrative therapeutic systems. With 18 books and over 300 professional and scientific articles to his credit, Dr. Lazarus is widely recognized as an international authority on effective and efficient psychotherapy. *The American Psychologist* (published monthly by the American Association of Psychology) had an article some years back of a survey in which Professor Lazarus was listed as one of the 10 most influential psychotherapists of the twentieth century.

Allen Fay, M.D., is the Associate Clinical Professor of Psychiatry at the Mount Sinai School of Medicine in New York. He received his medical degree from New York Medical College and was trained in psychiatry at New York's Mount Sinai Hospital. He is a Diplomate of the American Board of Psychiatry and Neurology, and has practiced psychiatry in New York for 35 years. He teaches cognitive-behavioral approaches to therapy at the Mount Sinai School of Medicine. In 1999, the psychiatry residents named him Teacher of the Year. Dr. Fay is the author of *Making Things Better By Making Them Worse, The Invisible Diet, Making It As A Couple, I Can If I Want To* (with Arnold Lazarus), and *Don't Believe It For A Minute* (with Arnold Lazarus and Clifford Lazarus).

> *Chapunoff:* Arnold and Allen, I'd like to ask you first about the marital dispute I described in Chapter 11, between "Bob and Mary." If you had seen this couple in consultation, how would you have approached the situation?

Fay: Ed, one could write a chapter just on that interaction. One of the first things I would do is to use the material they present as an opportunity to practice in the office better ways of communicating. A major point I make in the book Making It As A Couple is that style precedes content. That is, if people talk in a way that is not aggressive, not punitive, but supportive and collaborative, it enables their partners to listen to the message. On the other hand, if the style is confrontational, the partner is going to get defensive and the problems will not be addressed, let alone resolved.

You want to use the time you have with them as a practice session. They should be encouraged to talk to each other that way at every opportunity. In addition, it is important for them to practice the same thing outside the office. Sometimes, I recommend the use of a tape recorder at home. When they are communicating about topics that may be charged, they can turn the machine on and it will serve as a monitor. This technique will help them have better control of the conversation. They can then listen to the tape, not with the purpose of catching each other in a mistake, but to see what they can improve upon.

One of the basic principles of therapy and relationships in general is that when you see something positive, you reinforce and support it. So, when Mary says, "I want you to recover," you pick up on that rather than on her complaining. When she complains, you want to get her to say what she feels in a more constructive way.

Example: Instead of saying "I want you to pay more attention to me, for a change," Mary would say: "Bob, I'd like us to have more intimacy." You're modeling better communication. Asking for what you want in a pleasantly assertive way is better than complaining or criticizing.

It is important when talking about sexual problems to know whether the dissatisfaction is primary or secondary. Are these people who were never satisfied (primary sexual problem)? Or was their relationship wonderful at one time and then deteriorated (secondary sexual problem)? Although it is certainly possible to work with primary dysfunction or dissatisfaction, it's often easier to deal with a relationship (and sex life) that was previously satisfactory.

It is highly desirable for Bob and Mary to develop a better sense of empathy. Empathy is enormously important. Does Bob have a sense of what it is like to live the way Mary has with this deprivation for so many years? Is there anything he can think of that might be inhibiting his desire? Is he interested in continuing with the marriage and having a better sex life? If he thinks his marriage is viable, what ideas does he have to make it better?

With respect to Mary, it sounds as if she has passively accepted the situation with periodic complaints and outbursts rather than being assertive—that is, solution-oriented and collaborative.

We always explain to people the difference between unassertiveness, assertiveness, and aggressiveness. Assertiveness involves the capacity to ask for what you want without putting the other person down. Unassertiveness means that either you don't bring up a subject that concerns you, or, if you bring it up, you do so very indirectly and/or with a lot of guilt or anxiety. Aggressiveness means that you bring it up in a way that assaults the other person and doesn't respect his or her feelings. With this couple, Mary's aggressive and Bob's defensive. He clearly has deficiencies in assertiveness. It appears, however, that both have some capacity to respond to each other.

One should also find out if during this sexual drought, they enjoyed any kind of physical closeness, such as hugging or cuddling—in bed or out of bed.

Later in the visit, you mention that Mary feels that Bob has always thought that sex is dirty. If that's true, where did he get this notion? Did he ever have any positive sexual experience? Did he enjoy any kind of sexual contact? Is it intercourse that bothers him? Is it oral sex or sex during the menstrual period? Did he ever masturbate outside the relationship or within the relationship? Were there any other women in his life before they married? Is there anything in her style or physically that has been inhibiting him?

One of the sad facts is that there are millions of people whose relationships and sex lives are unsatisfactory, but who never get counseling. This is a couple that could probably benefit from therapy, and the outlook could be more favorable than it seems. It's just that they haven't had help, let alone the right kind of help.

Lazarus: I would have proceeded very much the way you did, and then I would have stressed the need to focus on three elements—his, her, and their issues. I might have come on a bit more forcefully and told them that given the way they miscommunicate, and in light of the years of anger, fears, and resentments that seem to exist, unless they made specific changes, the prognosis would not be at all favorable. I would explain that the acquisition of simple and straightforward skills could turn their lives around for the better. They would be told that they need to acquire proficiency in two main areas: communication skills and sexual skills. I would also add that Bob needs to change his outlook on sex.

In couples' therapy, I find it important for the therapist to convey that he or she is impartial and has no vested interest in saving the marriage. In fact, in some instances, the best and indeed the most positive outcome is to end an unhappy marriage as amicably as possible. Bob and Mary need to be informed that if they genuinely wish to remain married and are willing to put the effort into making certain changes, they will be given all the help and encouragement that the therapist can muster.

For a therapist to offer empathy, display good listening skills, and clarify the essence of a couple's specific problems is a good beginning. However, if training, feedback, coaching, guidance, and instruction are not also provided, it is my opinion that the patients are being shortchanged. In the case of Bob and Mary, they would only be wasting their time and money unless their therapist taught them exactly how to communicate effectively and enabled them to accept their respective entitlements. And when sexual problems are present, I think it is imperative for the therapist to discuss every nuance in an explicit and straightforward manner with no hesitations or any sense of embarrassment.

Chapunoff: Unfortunately, the best therapists and books on relationships are sometimes unable to avoid a divorce, which, incidentally, may not only be inevitable, but necessary. Do you ever recommend a permanent break in a couple's relationship, or just offer it as a viable option?

Fay: It is true that under the best circumstances (therapy and a high degree of motivation), some relationships are simply not viable. Despite our best efforts, some couples just don't make it. There are certain intrinsic fundamental incompatibilities. For example, one person absolutely does not want children, and the other requires children for fulfillment. They might have started their relationship with the mistaken belief that they could work this out.

There are also some "baggage" problems that may be insoluble. Some families, for instance, exert control and are intrusive. This leads to divided loyalties that make it difficult for relationships to survive. And there are many other things—major financial pressures or untreated psychiatric illnesses—that make it difficult for people to relate to each other.

There are those who continue to live together being miserable. I generally don't recommend that people break up. I tell them that my goal is to improve the quality of their relationship. If, in fact, there is some degree of caring for each other, it could be satisfying to stay together. But if they don't make it, the work they put into this relationship will enhance their individual ability to relate in the future. I think it's a mistake for a therapist to invest too much in people staying together, either because they are truly incompatible or because some couples will feel pressured and not respond well.

I am always pleased when people get along better. Whether they stay together or not is a secondary issue for me, unless there are young children involved, in which case it will be particularly important for them to get along better, and if possible, stay together.

Lazarus: If I consider a marriage emotionally bankrupt, I tend to share my feelings and impressions with the couple. I tell them that it is my professional opinion that an amicable divorce would be better than the hostility with which they live. I tend to recommend that they get a second opinion before heading to divorce lawyers. I have on several occasions offered my services to help couples part harmoniously (especially when young children have been in the picture), and on these occasions my "couples therapy" became "divorce counseling." About 2 years ago, I saw a couple in their forties where the wife said to her husband in my office, "I feel nothing but contempt for you." I determined that this statement was not blurted out in anger or said in temper, but that she truly meant it. I then pointed out how miserable it was for both of them to live under such conditions and recommended a parting of the ways. Instead, they went to another therapist (a former student of mine) who kept them in therapy until a few months ago, before they all concluded that divorce was the best option.

I have often said to my students and postdoctoral trainees, "If saving a marriage is more important to you than it is to the couple you are treating, it's time to take a good, hard look at yourself." It is my view that the message, "We must try to salvage this marriage at all costs" may tend to make couples more oppositional. On the other hand, I have found that if a couple engages in combative tactics in my office and I say, in a matter-of-fact tone, "Perhaps divorce would be a good option," this often shocks them into changing their ways and cooperating with the treatment plan.

Chapunoff: Arnold, in Making It as a Couple, Allen says that most relationships don't work. What is your view?

Lazarus: We obviously have no hard data to determine how many marriages really work, but given the divorce rate (more than 50 percent) we can infer that the majority do not fare too well. One may assume that of the 50 percent who remain together, many do so not because the relationship is working and they are happy, but out of fear, religious convictions, monetary considerations, and so forth. In my book Marital Myths Revisited, I state: "Most people don't know how to be married." So, I agree with Allen that most relationships don't work.

Chapunoff: Allen, do you have any comments on this?

Fay: Ed, when you take into account the number of divorces (not to mention the break-up rate in non-marriage relationships), as well as the number of people who live together feeling chronically unhappy or unfulfilled, it seems clear that in some sense or another, their relationships are not working. They are certainly not working as well as they could.

Chapunoff: Most people can afford a book dealing with intimate relationships, but not everybody is able to pay a psychiatrist or a psychologist. If distressed couples followed your advice, what percentage of them do you estimate could benefit substantially?

Lazarus: My estimate is about half of them would derive significant help—that is, if they manage to extricate themselves from a dreadful marriage, or they are able to turn things around so that they give and receive the love and support they desire. And I would add that if this has not occurred within 5 to 10 sessions, it is unlikely to happen even after months or years of therapy or counseling.

One of the chief drawbacks is when one or both partners have severe problems. To be married to a person with, for example, an obsessive–compulsive disorder, major recurring depressions, or a borderline or narcissistic personality, it will likely derail the relationship. Even the best therapists may be unable to make headway. Let's not forget the fact that patients may show up for therapy without really wanting to be helped. I have seen quite a number of couples wherein one of the spouses was present simply to be able to say, "Well, I did my best to save this marriage. I even went for counseling." In fact, with one couple I saw very recently, I worked hard to help them improve their relationship, only to learn, in the end, that the wife was seriously in love with another man (about whom her husband was completely unaware). She had come to see me only to placate her parents who knew about the affair, and who had insisted that she receive professional help for her marriage in the hope that this would change her mind.

Fay: It is certainly true that many people can't afford psychotherapy, although there are many facilities that offer flexible or reduced fees. There are some research programs where there is no fee, and this also applies to couples' therapy. Some university psychology departments offer this.

155

Most couples who get therapy get some benefit from it. How much benefit they get depends on a number if issues. Are there absolute, major, irreconcilable, non–negotiable incompatibilities? How heavy is the biological loading? How motivated are they to improve the relationship? Do both partners display goodwill and good faith? It is also important to determine how serious the pressures of reality are: Is a partner or child seriously or chronically ill? Are there major financial constraints? Are there meddlesome and disruptive family influences? Often, people just need information or simple exercises to turn things around.

The majority of couples who come to therapy genuinely want to get along better. If they are willing to work at it, practice some exercises at home, or get the right kind of therapy, a significant number of them will benefit. And it doesn't necessarily take a long time either. Some people benefit from one session, two sessions, or ten sessions. I've seen a few couples for a number of years, but most who come for a few visits get something out of it, particularly in conjunction with some reading, listening to tapes, or specific exercises.

Lazarus: I certainly agree with Allen, but I would like to point out that we have all seen couples who come in looking as if they are in serious trouble because of all the clashing, cursing, and colliding that goes on, and yet, after a while, it becomes clear that this was all hot air. With some sensible relationship prescriptions, they drop the phony war and settle down into a loving relationship.

Chapunoff: In established relationships (normal or dysfunctional), do you find that couples usually "express" more than they "repress," or is it the other way around? Some people keep a marriage going despite voicing frequent discontent and unhappiness. The partners honestly tell each other the way it is, and almost never have a peaceful day—let alone a peaceful night.

Others keep quiet, resent the relationship, and hate their mate's guts, but you never hear a discussion or an argument between them. If it isn't too ridiculous a question, can you tell me which behavior is more dysfunctional?

Lazarus: I know of no studies that have shown how many couples express and how many repress their feelings. There are those who believe that "repressors" who internalize their discontent and do not vent it will damage their health. Of course, in all the cases we see in our offices, at least one of the partners has expressed discontent, or they would not be there. Thus, they have a chance to make things better. Those who remain silent seem destined to suffer in silence. Nevertheless, it is important to note that the field of psychotherapy has made a 180-degree shift away from the quintessential "let it all hang out" philosophy. While under the domination of Freudian thinking, where mental and emotional well-being was supposed to rest on the putative value of getting in touch with and expressing virtually all one's significant thoughts and feelings, repression was seen as the cause of much suffering.

Current thinking is that there are many issues that are best ignored, forgotten, and not expressed. Therefore, the important question that must be addressed is which events, feelings, issues are better dealt with and openly expressed, and which ones should be kept to oneself. It is the therapist's task to help a patient determine when keeping quiet will prove unproductive, and when speaking up is necessary (and vice versa). Of course, anything taken to an extreme will probably have adverse consequences. Thus, as you implied, those couples who feel that they must vent everything, and who enter tedious discussions and often argue right through the night, are merely asking for trouble. On the other hand, when someone suppresses and holds in a fierce and deep-seated grudge, and is seething with unexpressed resentment, this will obviously undermine the quality of the relationship. As Allen explained, it is in this situation where the therapist can help that person express him- or herself in a way that will not aggravate matters but will likely alleviate the situation.

Fay: We are again dealing with the fundamental issue of assertiveness, and to what extent people have the capacity to control their emotions, especially negative emotions.

In the first book we did together, I Can If I Want To, Arnie and I took the position that it was a mistake to encourage people to express anger as anger. That was a time when the vast majority of therapists thought that it was healthy to let the anger out. The point is not whether you express or repress feelings, but how you express them. The overt expression of anger in intimate relationships, in my opinion, is almost always destructive, although in otherwise solid relationships, occasional expressions of anger are often tolerated quite well.

There are many things we overlook in relationships in order to make them work: dissatisfactions, disappointments, and frustrations. It isn't necessary to verbalize everything that is on your mind. However, it is important to request things that are essential to you, such as certain changes in your partner's behavior. Again, the critical issue is how you express what you want. Changes should be requested about important things. If the issue is minor, generally it's better to let it pass.

One of the best predictors of the quality of a relationship is the capacity to tolerate differences of opinion and differences in style and habits. There are countless differences between partners in a relationship, and if you made an issue about every single one, there wouldn't be time for anything else.

So, I think that people who live happily together strike a balance between what they express and what they let pass. If one of the partners comments on his or her dissatisfaction, he or she could say: "I'd really like to do something about our sex life. Maybe the doctor can help us." That's a lot better than the things people often say to each other in relationships, such as: "We never have sex;" "You always rejected me;" "You're just like your father/mother; it's no wonder you don't want sex; your parents haven't had sex for thirty years;" or "You're always making excuses."

Accusations or criticisms don't contribute to solving the problem. Doing the opposite will. Words or gestures must be expressed in a non-threatening way. If a person feels assaulted, he or she may become defensive or withdrawn.

Getting back to Bob and Mary: Here you have a woman who is suffering and has been suffering for a long time. She is frustrated and has tried many different things that haven't worked. This couple, like many others, would like to be happier and just don't know how. And that's one of the main purposes of reading a book or going to a therapist.

Chapunoff: There are many relationship traps (e.g. complaining, making negative predictions, exploiting your partner's weakness, making unilateral decisions, lying, making excuses, giving orders, and so on). Multiple conflicts and disagreements appear to be the rule, rather than the exception. Have you noticed that when three or four of them are corrected, the remaining traps have a much better chance for a permanent solution, or do some of the conflicts remain stubbornly unresolved?

Lazarus: There is often a positive snowball effect, especially when a couple's problems revolve around similar traps. Thus, if a couple who resorts to criticism, disapproval, blaming, complaining, and dredging up past mistakes learns to be less critical, all of these issues often fall into place. But there are other traps that prove stubborn. In my experience, it is often most difficult to put an end to jealousy and dishonesty.

Fay: Many years ago, a colleague of mine at Mount Sinai, Dr. Louis Linn, referred to the ripple effect, that is, the idea that change in one area often spreads to other areas even if those areas are not specifically addressed. Psychologists call it generalization. It is true that when people successfully address a few of the problem areas, the overall quality of the relationship often improves significantly, and the other traps seem less important, or they actually become less obvious.

Chapunoff: Is attitude a function of character? If it is, does this explain why people's attitudes are so difficult to change, if we consider that character traits are carried for a lifetime?

Lazarus: Character—implying one's basic and fundamental makeup—will certainly exert an impact on the way one responds to and views the world (meaning one's attitudes). About 50 years ago, American psychology focused on the impact of an individual's environment. There was a widespread view that most things could be modified. Today, the pendulum has swung in the opposite direction as more and more evidence has come to light about the impact of genetic and constitutional factors. One's "hardwiring" places definite limitations on what can be changed.

Your question about "character traits" being carried throughout one's life is most important. I think that "temperament" is tied to what you have called "character traits." And the evidence points to the fact that this is inborn. We all know people with sweet, happy-go-lucky, laid-back, easygoing temperaments or personalities, and other people who are irascible, quick-tempered, testy, petulant, and hostile.

My opinion is that the concept of "thresholds" explains some of the underlying issues. If we think of someone who has a high pain-tolerance threshold, a high frustration-tolerance threshold, and a high stress-tolerance threshold, that person is likely to be a pleasant and easygoing individual. On the other hand, someone with low thresholds of this kind—especially low frustration-tolerance threshold—will, in common parlance, be a high maintenance partner or friend. Can one increase these thresholds? Yes, but only to a limited extent. Methods such as relaxation training, rational disputation, and assertiveness training might be of some help, as will the use of certain medications. But the person will be prone to suffer, blow up, and overdramatize minor events— and remain the type of individual we would hope our sons and daughters never marry.

Fay: A familiar saying in our culture is that "you can't teach an old dog new tricks." I've had enough experience doing therapy with older people to observe that people in the eighties and nineties can change very quickly if they are given the right tools and the right insights.

We were taught as psychiatry residents that we should not acquiesce to a patient's expectations of getting better in a short period. Yet, I find the opposite orientation to be helpful. I expect people to be better in a short period, and if they aren't, I try to see what it is that I am missing, either in my assessment of the problem or in my therapy.

This leads to an interesting discussion about the subject of resistance in psychotherapy. This may be a little far afield for this book, but many years ago, in a chapter that Arnie and I did for a book entitled Resistance, we took the position that the source of resistance to change in therapy was not in the patient but in the therapist and in the therapy. Although this isn't literally true in every case, we felt that it was important as an operating model. Thus, instead of assuming that a patient not improving is the result of factors within the patient, we operate on the premise that the failure to improve is more related to what we are doing or not doing. That way, we can look to ourselves to find more creative solutions to the patient's problems, which is why patients come to us in the first place.

Certain problems are not situational but are structurally built into the character and personality. They therefore often require a little more practice to overcome. Certain qualities of temperament require medication to achieve better regulation. People who are markedly hyper-reactive to relatively mild provocation often have the kind of dysregulation that cannot be corrected with psychotherapy alone. People with chronically explosive tempers or those who get hysterical over minor issues often benefit enormously from pharmacotherapy, which in turn enables them to benefit from psychotherapy. I certainly would not assume that because people have had something for a long time, either they cannot change, or will have great difficulty changing.

Chapunoff: A male child watches his father having an extramarital relationship for 3 decades with the full knowledge of his wife, and everyone else for that matter. The child, now an adult, hates his father because of what he did to the patient's mother and siblings, to the point that when the father dies, the son refuses to attend the funeral. But he marries, and then becomes engaged in the same kind of behavior (long-term extramarital relationship). Can you tell me why?

Fay: No, I can't tell you. There's an unscientific and illogical tendency in our field to make direct causal connections between past events and present events. It is certainly correct that we are the way we are because of biological factors, including our genes, as well as our lifetime of learning experiences. However, there are many people who see their parents doing all kinds of things, and they don't do them. They may even take strong stands against such behavior and live up to their own standards of conduct. So, it's important not to say that the young man engaged in such behavior because he saw his father do it.

Lazarus: The obvious thoughts that come to mind are modeling, example, and guilt, wherein his behavior would draw him closer to the father he so rejected. But without taking a full history, this would only be guesswork. Could it be a case where he hated his father for engaging in a behavior or temptation that he could sense within himself?

Fay: Ed, we have to look at the specific behavior and see what impact it has on a relationship. In some marriages, an extramarital relationship by one or both parties is the only thing that allows the couple to continue. There are some marriages where people get along very well, they are good friends, they are cooperative, they have many things in common, and they care a great deal about each other—but they are sexually incompatible in a way that is not amenable to therapy. There are other configurations as well. Whether I like it, you like it, or we don't like it, it's nevertheless a fact that some relationships would not be viable in a model of sexual exclusivity.

Chapunoff: There are many books on relationship conflicts and how to deal with them. I'd like to learn more about prevention. When I went to school, I was taught geography, history, mathematics, and the rest. No teacher ever discussed how to prepare yourself for the trip of your life, how to ride the marital rocket, and how to avoid a crash landing on the wrong planet.

Lazarus: This is not a question but a statement—with which I agree. I think there are now books on the market that people who intend to marry or live together can read for a roadmap of how best to function. A book in this area that I like is Sam Hamburg's Will Our Love Last? I have maintained for many years that our educational system fails to teach interpersonal skills in a proper, formal, well-thought-out way. In my book Marital Myths Revisited, I state that if high schools routinely offered courses in "marriage competence," it is likely that more people would know how to develop sensible, workable, and loving marriages. But I also ask, "Who would be qualified to teach these courses?"

Unfortunately, many marriage counselors, psychologists, psychiatrists, and other mental health practitioners labor under as many false conceptions as the clients they counsel or treat.

Fay: We are taught the full spectrum of academic courses in school, and while these subjects are of great importance in helping us to prepare for life's challenges, there's no set of skills that is more important for personal happiness than the ability to communicate effectively with other people, particularly in intimate relationships.

People who are highly motivated often just need information and some mechanisms to effect change. Few individuals are fortunate enough to learn this early in life from parents or other role models. Learning communication skills in school is probably the best preventive measure.

Chapunoff: Would you please give us your thoughts about being happy, being miserable, life in general, and relationships in particular?

Lazarus: This question is very broad. I think that the work of Albert Ellis has focused on this domain. He has books that show how one can manufacture misery by thinking irrationally, by being demanding, self-critical, and so forth.

Fay: I agree. The question is so broad that it's difficult to answer, but I think that much misery is self-inflicted by believing certain things that are indeed irrational or simply incorrect. People tend to be happy when they appreciate the things they have and have developed good communication skills; when they are not exquisitely sensitive and hyper-reactive to differences between themselves and their partners; when they know how to have friends, how to do the things they love to do to the greatest extent possible, and how to pursue their passions. Hardly anyone is perfect at this. Also, absence of severe economic hardship and other overwhelming sources of stress make it more possible to achieve a quality existence. Some people are even able to overcome such stresses by maintaining perspective and telling themselves things that are helpful and therapeutic. In fact, these are some of the major goals of therapy: to relieve specific symptoms and improve problem-solving skills.

Chapunoff: Allen and Arnold, you've shared with me and the readers, thoughts, concepts and conclusions that resulted from many years of hard work and fruitful experiences. You have granted me a very special privilege. I don't know how to thank you enough.

Fay: I found the questions important and challenging, and I was delighted to respond to them.

Lazarus: The questions you raised are excellent, and I hope that my answers will prove helpful. You have obviously thought hard and long and had a tremendous amount of experience with the subject matter you are covering in this excellent book. You really know what important issues need to be addressed. I thank you for including me in this project. I found my participation both challenging and extremely stimulating.

PART FOUR

WHAT YOU CAN DO

Chapter 13

Back to Bed: Rush versus Procrastination

Timing is so important that sometimes we can afford to do the wrong thing—when the timing is right.

The majority of doctors and patients avoid discussing the right time to resume sexual activity following a heart attack, an acute cardiac crisis, or cardiac surgery. It's a mutual repression—a subconscious, silent conspiracy, if you will—or at best, if we want to be benign about it, an inadvertent omission.

This lapse in patient–doctor communication often leads patients to make their own decisions, and these are not always the correct ones. Read what follows, and then you will understand precisely what I'm talking about.

Before we do that, a few words of caution. The timing for resumption of sexual activity is not determined by a book or general principles. It's true that this kind of information gives you an overall idea on when and how most cardiac patients are able to proceed. Nevertheless, your particular case is unique and should be treated by your healthcare practitioner accordingly. Use the general information you find here as a springboard to ask your healthcare provider specifically when you should resume sexual activity, and follow his/her advice.

PREMATURE SEXUAL ACTIVITY FOLLOWING A HEART ATTACK

PHYSICIAN: "You are telling me that you had sex without waiting for my recommendations, and so soon following your coronary? Walter, didn't you think it was risky?"

PATIENT: "No, I thought it was worthy!"

When John was about to celebrate his forty-eighth birthday, the cake had to wait for another occasion. He experienced an oppressive feeling in his chest and was hospitalized with an acute myocardial infarction. Three days later, when he was transferred out of the intensive care unit to a private room, he made a request: he wanted his wife to sleep in the same room. The hospital obliged with a cot.

John had a very happy marriage. His wife was totally devoted to him and invariably tried to please him in every possible way. Her former husband had been a violent man, so she truly appreciated John, who was "kind, generous, and considerate." The couple had been together for several years and enjoyed a prolific sex life.

A week following his heart attack, John asked himself some agonizing questions: Did my coronary finish me off? Am I impotent?

To lessen his doubts, he asked his wife to engage in some sexual play. She first refused, thinking (very logically, indeed) that it wasn't safe for him to do it. But he insisted and once more, the eternally agreeable and compliant wife, always ready to please him, consented.

It was the tenth day of hospitalization. (This incident took place years ago, when hospitalizations for acute myocardial infarctions were considerably longer than they currently are.)

They went into the bathroom. John sat on the toilet seat, put a couple of pillows behind his back, and his wife performed fellatio on him. According to John, he had a "fair erection and ejaculation." He also noted "no cardiac reactions," but felt tired and slept for about 8 hours without interruption. He related the incident to me one day before his discharge. He wanted reassurances that "nothing bad had happened" to his heart.

Several reasons may explain why John got away with his imprudence.

- ♥ The sex act only took a few minutes, and he watched for any possible discomforts, as he later explained.
- ♥ He avoided eating before the effort, which prevented an additional burden on his heart.
- ♥ The pillows behind his back gave him a very comfortable and relaxing position.
- ♥ A coronary angiogram done after John's heart attack showed that only one coronary artery (and not the most important one) was affected. The others were free of any blockages. So, his prospects for a full recovery were excellent.
- ♥ Last but not least, fellatio was his favorite pastime, next to stamp collecting.

I presume that cases like this one are unusual. The main concern of most patients who have had a recent heart attack is just to recover as soon as possible and resume a normal life. Besides, they are also psychologically vulnerable and physically debilitated. Still, as you can see, curiosity about the survival of sexual prowess may be strong enough to prevail.

If you are ever tempted to improvise in a similar way, however, please refrain. During the second week following an acute myocardial infarction, lighter sexual outlets should be contemplated (Chapter 14).

EXCESSIVE DELAY IN SEXUAL ACTIVITY FOLLOWING CORONARY BYPASS SURGERY

PHYSICIAN TO A PATIENT, A COUPLE OF MONTHS AFTER CARDIAC SURGERY: "Louis, are you ready to talk about sex?"

PATIENT: "No, I'm ready to do it!"

Just as some heart attack patients rush into sex too quickly, other patients go to the opposite extreme and wait an unnecessarily long time to initiate sex. Although there are many reasons for postponing sex, the heart itself (interestingly enough) is usually not the cause for procrastination.

About ⅔ of patients who undergo cardiac surgery leave the hospital without any counseling on sexuality. In one study, the average time for resumption of sexual activity by post-surgery cardiac patients was 5.7 weeks. Patients who had acute myocardial infarctions took longer: 9.4 weeks. Lack of information due to faulty patient–doctor communication may be responsible for long and unjustified delays.

Jean, a 40-year-old unhappily married woman, had cardiac surgery. For months following the operation, she continued to complain of severe chest pains and blamed these for her "inability" to have sexual relations with her husband. One day, she told me the chest pains did not exist and she had been "faking the discomfort" as an excuse to avoid intimacy. She accepted a consultation with a psychotherapist.

In the past several years, technical improvements in cardiac surgery have been impressive. Still, the patient has to deal with the uncertainty of his or her outcome, physical discomforts, complications that prolong a hospital stay, longer than expected recovery period, work and financial disruptions, family responsibilities, depression, anxiety, prohibition of smoking, less food, less alcohol, less salt, and less sex (at least for some time).

Doctor communication may be responsible for long and unjustified delays.

Philip and his wife, Laura, first consulted me several months following his coronary bypass surgery. Laura was in a "no-nonsense" mood.

Laura: "Ask the doctor, Phil, ask him."

Philip: "Ask him...what?"

Laura: "You know what. What's wrong with you? Are you getting senile?"

Philip: "Oh, I think I know what you mean. You're talking about sex, right?"

Laura: "Of course I'm talking about sex. What else could it be? After 5 months and 10 days without it, I don't think there's anything else we should be talking about.!"

Philip: "Darling, please, don't get upset..."

Laura: "Well, I'm sorry, but I can assure you—this time, I'm not going to leave the doctor's office without some answers."

This couple had never received any sexual counseling. Sex had been avoided for fear of doing something wrong or damaging. They believed that if the doctor didn't mention anything about sex, then they were not supposed to have it.

This vacuum of information causes upset and deception.

Low self-esteem due to extensive surgical scars may have its own impact, particularly in female patients. I've heard complaints about the "ugliness" of post-operative scars, even when the healing process was normal. The doctor, and especially the sexual partner, must provide encouragement by minimizing the negative effect of the scars on the patient's physical attractiveness.

A woman in her early forties revealed to me "how devastated" she was about the healing wounds she had between her breasts and on her leg and thigh. (The leg, thigh, or both, provide segments of veins that are harvested by the surgeon to be used as bypass grafts of the coronary arteries.) I was pressed to find a solution. Since we couldn't get rid of the scars, and in order to make them less visible, I advised her to wear a long negligee and sexy stockings. This turned out to be a blessing in disguise. The results were spectacular. Had it not been for the wounds, her husband might not have received a longtime wish: he had always wanted to see his wife in sexy undergarments, but he had been too bashful to ask.

Chapter 14

What to Do and When to Do It

PATIENT: "Doctor, I had a coronary three months ago, and my
 sex life has been bad!"

PHYSICIAN: "How was it prior to the heart attack?"

PATIENT: "Terrible!"

PHYSICIAN: "Well, I'm glad to know you're getting better!"

When the physician states it is safe to resume sex, he or she is
usually referring to intercourse. But is that all there is? Is sex
the exclusive act of intercourse? Of course not.

Intercourse, or coitus, is vaginal penetration by the penis.
However, sexual expression doesn't always mean vaginal penetration. Not at all. Although this may seem obvious, it is remarkable
how many people equate sex with intercourse. Because readiness for
sexual activity is an important element in the recovery process of a
cardiac illness, ignorance of the distinction between sex and intercourse can cause the patient and his or her sexual partner to miss
valuable moments of emotional and physical contact.

Sexual activity can be coital and non-coital. The patient may be
advised to have one type or another at different stages of the conva-

lescent period. The techniques available for intimacy should never make us neglect or underestimate the importance of a tender kiss, a sweet smile, or the warm touch of a hand.

Recommendations for resuming intimacy and sex should only be made on individual basis. All heart conditions are different, and so are the patients who experience them. What to do, when to do it, and how much to do, depends upon:

- The status of the cardiovascular system
- The general medical condition and presence of associated ailments
- The prescribed and non-prescribed (over-the-counter) medications being taken
- The psychological state of mind that preceded and followed the cardiac crisis
- The patient's and sexual partner's previous sexual performance
- The quality of the couple's relationship in general
- Individual concepts about sexuality

The first five points are self-explanatory. Let me give you examples of situations that deal with points six and seven.

The Quality of the Relationship

Two women had myocardial infarctions of similar severity, and both recovered well. One has a loving and caring husband, and the other suffers a terrible marriage—a nightmare for the past 20 years with a man who abuses her emotionally and physically. In fact, her heart attack occurred after a violent physical and verbal barrage.

The happy woman will be able to resume lovemaking in several weeks. I don't necessarily mean full sexual intercourse in a very short period of time, but delicate, gradual, truly loving physical contact, until she fully recovers.

The woman with the abusive husband won't be in the position to resume intimacy. She'll need immediate counseling, even before she goes home. She will have to avoid further contact with her husband and report the situation to the police. And she will need to learn how to handle situations that represent a threat to her security and her life.

Individual Concepts about Sexuality

Two men in their early fifties are recovering well from their respective heart attacks. One is open-minded and liberal in his sexual views. The other is not. Both express concern about the possibility of facing erection failure during the first attempt to make love after their myocardial infarctions.

The patient with a liberal attitude can be advised to try self-stimulation for several days before attempting to have regular intercourse. This does not have to end in orgasm or ejaculation. It's simply a preparatory exercise. It isn't too demanding, and it proves the presence (or absence) of an erection.

Counseling for the conservative patient must be approached differently; he's prudish and holds tightly to his rules on sexuality. Most likely, any suggestion of masturbation, even coming from the doctor as medical advice, will not be acceptable. Other options must be made available to him. He may be advised to get physically closer to his wife—avoiding intercourse until he recovers—and observe his erectile response.

The physical aspects of sexuality go hand in hand with spiritual and intellectual communication. This is a major foundation of any successful intimate relationship. Sharing books, movies, concerts, games, exhibits, lectures, conversations, picnics, and traveling—all contribute to the pursuit of a happy union.

The following guidelines use the post-heart attack (myocardial infarction) patient as a model. They can also assist those individuals who have any number of cardiac conditions. Remember: Your sexual activity should be planned according to your doctor's instructions. What follows here is only intended to give you a basic understanding of what is generally possible or acceptable to do.

Only your doctor should decide what is the proper thing for you to do. And don't forget that it may be very beneficial to invite your sexual partner to participate in these discussions.

A practical tip: If you have reservations about talking directly to your physician about sexual contact options, make photocopies of this chapter's general suggestions, show them to the physician, and inquire what is allowable and what it is not. He/she can make a mark in the paper and give you the needed information.

SEXUAL ACTIVITY FOLLOWING A HEART ATTACK OR OTHER CARDIAC CONDITION

Note: The guidelines below are not intended as recommendations for any cardiac patient's sexual activity. They are intended to assist you with ideas and suggestions. Only your physician can make decisions about appropriate options and timing for sexual activity.

Non-coital/Non-genital Sexual Activity (no vaginal penetration/no genital contact)

During the first and second week post-myocardial infarction (PMI), I recommend engaging in the activities listed below, not because they necessarily express sensuality, but because they promote closeness, affection, trust, and confidence. Perhaps most importantly, they are also a way to communicate love.

- Caressing
- Cuddling
- Holding
- Hugging
- Kissing
- Massaging
- Scratching
- Touching

Missing out on these various forms of contact deprives the couple of a number of physical, emotional, and psychological benefits. All of these physical expressions are very important, including scratching and massage. Properly done, they provide enormous relaxation and pleasure. If you never tried them, I urge you to start today. If your mate gets the idea correctly, and does it to you regularly, you'll realize how much you've been missing. These "touching" variations are welcome at any time, as soon as the very acute period of the illness is overcome and visits to the intensive care unit are allowed.

Non-coital/Genital Sexual Activity (no vaginal penetration/genital contact) and Coital Sexual Activity (vaginal penetration)

Most physicians recommend that sex be avoided for 6 to 8 weeks after an acute myocardial infarction. This recommendation usually includes non-coital activity with significant excitement (e.g. oral–genital sex), as well as coital activity (with vaginal penetration).

Myocardial infarctions vary in severity. Additionally, complications and recovery times depend on many extra-cardiac factors, including other illnesses, psychological and emotional issues, and the quality of the patient and partner's relationship. Therefore, each patient needs individual assessment when it comes to resuming sexual activity. Your physician should advise you when to have sexual contact and, if possible, be specific about any positions that could help you or hurt you. Some recoveries from myocardial infarctions go so smoothly and satisfactorily that sex may be tried during the third or fourth week PMI. Taking a post-myocardial infarction stress test is both useful and reassuring before deciding when to resume sex.

SOME PRACTICAL ASPECTS OF SEXUAL CONTACT
Manual Genital Stimulation
Manual genital stimulation between partners, and engaging in self-stimulation, is part of the search for erotic sensations. When the experience has a positive impact, it results in arousal, sexual pleasure, or both.

It generally requires less effort for the cardiac convalescent to stimulate his or her partner than being stimulated. There are exceptions: If a patient stimulates a partner who takes too long to react, or is too demanding, the involvement can be very taxing.

Conclusion: It isn't non-coital or coital sex that necessarily defines the degree of energy and effort that will be involved in the sexual act. A good deal depends on the partners' personalities, flexibility, cooperation, and understanding.

Oral–Genital Sex
Fellatio for men and cunnilingus for women can also induce or augment sexual arousal or lead to orgasm. Stimulation can be done from one partner to the other, or it can be carried out simultaneously. This latter technique is called "69." With a little imagination, the inverted position of the couple resembles that number.

A female cardiac convalescent can perform fellatio by positioning herself at the side of her partner, either in a kneeling position or lying down, with her body oriented toward her partner.

A male cardiac convalescent can perform cunnilingus in the following undemanding way: While the female lies in bed, her husband (the patient), kneels on a pillow placed on the floor and embraces her hips with his arms, then proceeds with oral-genital contact. This position demands minimal effort because the patient's arms are totally relaxed, resting on the bed. It is particularly recommended for convalescent patients whose partners achieve gratification and orgasms without the need of vaginal thrusting. This latter maneuver requires a greater effort, regardless of whether the patient is a man or a woman.

Coital Sex

WIFE: "Fred, what's your favorite position?"

HUSBAND: "Any one that doesn't give you a headache, darling!"

In general, cardiac patients are advised to continue using the same coital positions they have enjoyed for many years. It can be difficult for some people to adopt new ones. Nevertheless, sometimes new positions may need to be considered and viewed with an open mind, particularly when they are medically beneficial.

Let's first review the most important positions, and then I'll make a few comments for special situations.

Man on Top, Partners Face-to-Face

This is the most common position used in the United States. It's also called the missionary position. Cardiac patients who lie flat on their backs should avoid the weight of their partners on their chest because that creates a significant burden. If the patient is on top, the hands are pressed against the bed and the upper extremities are somewhat stiff for a while. That increases the workload of the heart, at times, beyond desirable levels.

Those who have had heart failure or have "a weak pump" due to coronary artery disease, valvular heart disease, cardiomyopathies, or other causes, experience shortness of breath when lying down. In this position, the lungs are more congested than when the chest is vertically oriented. Placing several pillows behind the back helps.

These observations do not mean that the missionary position should be avoided, but cardiac convalescents should be aware of the potential problems described and make the necessary adjustments and corrections.

Woman on Top, Partners Face-to-Face

This position is also very popular, and offers more control of sexual movement for the woman. If the woman is on top, the man, of course, is at the bottom. This is not what many men prefer, as they see themselves as acting too passively, or in a subdued or unmasculine manner.

Side to Side, Face-to-Face

Here the partners face each other lying on their sides. This is a relaxed position in that it avoids the burden of the other person's weight. The introduction of the penis into the vagina is not as easy in this position, particularly when the erection isn't strong. The couple can solve this problem by the vaginal introduction of the penis in missionary position and then rolling over onto the side.

Some cardiac patients notice discomfort (pounding, palpitations, or chest tightness), when lying on their left side. This is because the heart gets closer to the wall of the thoracic cage (chest wall), and that limits its motion, causing some strain. Lying on the right side or on the back can prevent these unpleasant symptoms.

Rear Entry

In this position, the man places the penis into the vagina from behind, as he faces the woman's back. This can be done with the woman on her hands and knees, and also in sitting and standing positions.

Patients who have had recent cardiac surgery and have a sore chest wound will benefit from this position because direct contact with the sensitive thorax will be avoided. In some cases, this chest area remains painful to the touch for several months following the operation. In general, cardiac patients also find this position helpful because breathing is easier than when lying flat.

Anal Intercourse

This form of intercourse may be demanding, particularly when the anal sphincter (anal muscle) is too tight. Acceptability of this position also depends on the overall status of the heart, blood pressure, heart rate, and rhythm abnormalities. Easy access to anal penetration is of great importance because the maneuver can be painful when the anal ring is not compliant. Generous lubrication facilitates introduction. Distention of a noncompliant anus may cause circulatory system reflexes that lower the blood pressure and slow the heart rate to levels that may not be tolerated. Dizziness and fainting could result in those whose blood pressure suddenly drops significantly. For example, a systolic blood pressure of 140 mm Hg that abruptly falls to 65 mm Hg may lead to a syncopal attack (blackout spell).

CONCLUSION

Positions and methods of sexual interaction considered beautiful by some, may be viewed as disgusting and forbidden by others. Compliance with a partner's desires may be difficult or impossible because of differences in taste, cultural background, or the emotional impact of a past or present relationship. However, indifference to a sexual partner's desires is an open invitation to trouble.

More than ever before, this is your time to develop the ability to listen, the flexibility to change, and the capacity to reprogram your mind and the marital relationship in the right direction. Relegate past errors to the past. Now you have an opportunity to learn and improve. Use it to the best of your ability and be grateful for having been granted another opportunity to become a little wiser, a better husband or wife—and why not a better lover as well.

Chapter 15

Erectile Dysfunction and the Heart

HUSBAND: "Darling, my cardiologist says it's okay for us to have sex."

WIFE: "That's great. Just make sure you double-check it with your psychologist."

Recognizing the existence of a problem is the first step toward solving it. Primary care physicians and cardiologists are not trained to treat sexual dysfunctions (SD) that result from emotional/psychological conflicts. Never try to convert these doctors into psychiatrists, psychologists, or sex therapists. They are not.

One thing your doctor can do—and I think he or she *should* do—is listen attentively to the description of your problem. I suggest you ask your physician if he or she would be receptive to answering some questions concerning your sexual dysfunction. If the physician answers affirmatively, describe your problem without ambiguities. Be as focused and direct as possible. If the physician has the answer, he or she will give it to you. If not, ask him or her who could help you. If your doctor can't recommend anyone, do your own search. Contact other professionals or professional associations and people you know and trust. Review any prospective consultant's credentials, education and training background, and his or her reputation through the county medical association, institutions, or hospitals he or she is associated with.

ERECTILE DYSFUNCTION: HOW PREVALENT IS IT?

Erectile dysfunction (ED) is the inability to obtain and/or maintain penile erection sufficient for vaginal penetration and satisfactory intercourse.

Alfred C. Kinsey (1894–1956), a zoologist at Indiana University, pioneered statistical research on this subject, and in 1948 he published *Sexual Behavior in the Human Male*. He estimated that ED affected 2 percent of men at age 40, and 30 percent of men at age 70. In 1994, The Massachusetts Male Aging Study applied strict scientific methods to this same subject, and reported that over 50 percent of all men between 40 and 70 years of age have varying degrees of ED. It is currently estimated that 30 million men in the United States suffer from ED.

Past History Data that Suggest a Psychogenic (Psychological) Cause for Erectile Dysfunction (ED)

- Morning erections (about two a week)
- Spontaneous erections
- Erections induced by reading sexually explicit material
- Erections that occur with one partner but do not occur with another
- Masturbation-induced erections
- Erections produced during foreplay
- Abrupt onset of poor erections associated with personal or social stress (separation, divorce, affair, illness in the family, financial losses, job termination, and/or new/difficult job)

Human sexuality researchers William Masters and Virginia Johnson (authors of *Human Sexual Response,* 1966, and *Human Sexual Inadequacy,* 1970) believed that 90 percent of ED had a psychological origin. Most recently, it has been suggested that among all cases of impotence, 50 percent are physical and 50 percent are psychological. The purpose of a medical work-up is to identify all possible causes. Then, a treatment plan is prepared.

The methods used to treat ED are indirect and direct.

Indirect methods are based on the patient's mental/emotional condition as well as on sexual experience (behavioral) modifications. When the therapeutic action is exercised on the penis itself, the method of intervention is defined as direct. Let's first look at indirect methods.

INDIRECT METHODS OF INTERVENTION FOR ED
Psychotherapy
Psychotherapy aims at the correction of dysfunctional thoughts, behaviors, and sexual interactions that inhibit sexual stimulation and performance. The ideal treatment is one that achieves the maximum degree of success with a minimal amount of interventions. Treatment is often remarkably helped by the involvement of the sexual partner as well.

Freudian Psychoanalysis
In the United States, from the beginning of the twentieth century until the end of World War II, there was a strong emphasis on using Freudian principles of psychoanalysis to deal with sexual dysfunctions (SD).

The psychoanalytic (Freudian) approach has some important drawbacks for the resolution of ED. Too much emphasis is placed on the effects of unconscious conflicts in relation to the present conflicts of the relationship. Treatment may take years before the erection failure is resolved. Classical psychoanalysis involves intensive, long-term and frequent therapy sessions (often several times a week). Psychoanalysis has not been noticeably effective (particularly in the short term) in the treatment of this condition.

Cognitive–Behavioral Treatment

Another method is called cognitive–behavioral treatment. Cognitive factors that affect erections include persistent erroneous beliefs and assumptions about sexual performance. The patient internalizes his or her dysfunctional cognitions. For example, in the case of a man with poor erections, he may say to himself: *I'm not attractive. She will not like me. She'll think that my erections are always too soft. I'll never be able to make her happy.* Once these thoughts are identified, the therapist finds a specific way of dealing with them.

Proponents of behavioral therapy see sexual activity as a set of behaviors that can be modified by behavioral interventions. New lovemaking strategies and resources are implemented: sexual positions, relaxation techniques, assertiveness skills training, and sex education are all relevant in setting a new tone to the intimate experience.

The goal of cognitive–behavioral therapy is to generate a sense of trust between the couple and eliminate the fear of failure.

The efficacy of cognitive–behavioral sex therapy is quite well established for erectile difficulties.

DIRECT METHODS OF INTERVENTION FOR ED
Oral Treatments
Viagra, Levitra, and Cialis have made a very significant difference in the treatment of ED. These medications have become the easiest and

most practical method to deal with this condition. I discuss these drugs separately in much greater detail later in this chapter.

Herbs. The difference between herbs and drugs is that herbs have not been studied with extensive randomized testing as drugs have been. Therefore, their efficacy and the incidence of potential side effects is unknown. Consequently, we cannot recommend them. Such herbs include damiana, dong quai, sarsaparilla, pygeum, ginkgo biloba, ginseng, dehydroepiandrosterone (DHEA), royal jelly, l-arginine, ma huang, muira puama, and ephedrine. Saw palmetto is a popular herb that is effective in shrinking prostates, but men should exercise great caution using it because it will reduce the ejaculate volume when taken for long periods. There are more products of this kind not listed here.

Yohimbine. Yohimbine is obtained from the bark of a South American tree. There are some reports of successful use in treating erectile dysfunction of psychological origin. Yohimbine has to be taken three times a day. Side effects such as dizziness and headaches are frequent, and the drug should be avoided in patients who suffer from cardiovascular disease.

Trazadone. This older antidepressant has been associated with erections when taken in dosages of 50 mg, three times a day. A major side effect is sedation.

Apomorphine and other topical agents. Apomorphine and other agents that can be applied locally are currently under investigation.

Apomorphine is not an opiate. Its formula does not contain any morphine at all. In fact, morphine is a sedative, and apomorphine is a stimulant. The drug is used to treat patients suffering from Parkinson's disease. It was observed that many patients taking this medication had erections.

The drug has been medically known since 1869. A sublingual (tablet under the tongue) preparation has recently been developed that appears to be effective and safe. It produces penile erection by stimulating areas in the hypothalamus from where the stimulation moves downwards toward the spinal cord center for penile erection. The drug is also promising for treatment of sexual dysfunction in women.

For thousands of years, Man has tried numerous compounds to stimulate erections, including rhinoceros horns, snake venom, and snake blood, among others. The consequences were the decimation of rhinos and not much effect on erections. So, we go back to the Viagra, Levitra, and Cialis (PDE-5 inhibitors) option. However, other alternatives should be considered when:

- Patients do not respond to PDE-5 inhibitors.
- These drugs are contraindicated.
- Men who take it have significant side effects (headaches, for example).

Vacuum Erection Device

The vacuum erection device (VED) is a mechanical way of producing an erection. It may be effective with physical or psychological erection failures. Literature reports that 80 to 90 percent of patients have satisfactory results.

The VED consists of a vacuum chamber, a vacuum pump, and a constrictor device that is applied to the base of the shaft of the penis. This may be an elastic band, an O-ring, or a disc. The vacuum chamber is made of transparent plastic, in a length and diameter that will accommodate penises of different shapes and sizes.

An Austrian doctor, Otto Lederer, was the one who introduced the first VED design, and he got a U.S. patent for it in 1917. For several decades the device was largely ignored. The FDA approved the VED in

1982. In 1986, the first scientific article was published about it and made the device popular. In 1991, 40,000 VED were sold in the United States.

The VED is simple. One end of the vacuum chamber is open and must be of a size that allows the tumescent penis to fill it completely. The most commonly required inside diameters are 4.14 cm, 4.45 cm, and 4.76 cm (1 5/8, 1 3/4, and 1 7/8 inches). The mechanical pump is usually electric or hand operated. The penis is placed in the chamber and a vacuum is applied for 6 minutes. Improved penile rigidity may result from applying the vacuum for 1 to 2 minutes, then releasing the vacuum momentarily, and then reapplying it for another 3 to 4 minutes.

To keep the penis rigid when the vacuum is released, an elastic ring or band is applied to the base of the penis. This must be tight enough to maintain penis rigidity, but not too tight as to injure the penis. People who are taking aspirin or anticoagulant drugs may have local hematomas resulting from this maneuver. Additionally, the hair trapped by the elastic band may at times produce some discomfort. The constriction required to maintain penis rigidity can safely be applied for 30 minutes. The mechanism by which VED leads to an erection is by increased arterial blood flow to the penis during the vacuum effect. Maintenance of the erection is achieved by prolonged venous congestion resulting from the effect of the constricting band.

The bruises on the skin of the penis seen in patients who are on aspirin or anticoagulant drugs are painless and disappear within 48 hours. Hematomas may take longer to resolve, but have not caused problems.

Vacuum pressure should exceed 100 mm Hg but negative pressures beyond 180 mm Hg are unnecessary and can cause bruises. The VED should have a safety valve to control this pressure. If the VED does not have a safety valve, avoid using it.

Before purchasing a VED, the patient and his partner should look at a video and have a demonstration and teaching session.

The erection produced by the VED is different from spontaneous erections. The temperature of the penis is cooler than normal body temperature. Since the tumescence begins at the constricting band, the penis pivots at the base, which sometimes requires manual insertion of the penis into the vagina.

Some patients suffer from "performance anxiety," which is the main reason for their erectile difficulties. In these cases, the VED may provide a sense of security. If an erection is not achieved during foreplay, the VED can be used.

The device causes some loss of spontaneity during lovemaking. For those who have new partners and want to keep the sexual dysfunction to themselves, the VED is a bit cumbersome and difficult to conceal.

MUSE (Medicated Urethral System for Erection)

MUSE (alprostadil) is a small pellet inserted into the urethra. Burning pain occurs in 13 percent of patients who use it. The erection usually appears in 5 to 10 minutes and lasts for 30 to 60 minutes. The pellet should not be inserted more than once in 24 hours. Massaging the penis increases the response to the medication. Oral sex is not recommended because of documented severe allergic reactions caused by the drug.

Intrapenile Injection of Vasodilators

Like many accidental discoveries in medicine, such as what happened with penicillin and Viagra, among many others, the effect of vasodilators in inducing erections was a fortuitous incident.

In 1982, Ronal Virag, M.D., was performing vascular surgery that involved repairing lower extremity arteries. During the operation, he injected papaverine into a pelvic artery to prevent spasm in branches of the artery he was repairing. Branches of this artery (called the hypogastric artery) supply blood to the penis. Dr. Virag noted an unexpected phenomenon: a penis erection. So, he correctly concluded that papaverine was responsible for the erection. His observation meant the beginning of a new era in the treatment of ED.

A British physician, Giles Brindley, M.D., dropped his trousers at the American Urological Association annual meeting in 1983. With one hand he grabbed his penis, and with the other he injected into it a vasodilator called phentolamine. This produced an erection. The experiment took place in front of an amazed—and amused—medical audience. His discovery—and bold demonstration—earned him a rightful place in the history of penile erection and its therapy.

As has happened with early enthusiasm with many discoveries, the results of intra-penile injection of vasodilators were tempered by reality. Sometimes, these caused scarring of the penis. Additionally, painful erections occasionally occurred, which lasted over 4 hours (called "priapism"). They did not recede spontaneously, and emergent surgical "decompression" of the penis was required.

Other problems were seen as well. The patient (and often the sexual partner) had decreased sexual desire and arousal. The partner felt particularly affected because of presumption that the sexual act was "only consummated" because of the intra-penile injection-caused erection, and not because of physical attraction.

Still, this method, like any other available method to treat ED, is useful in selective cases. It requires education, awareness about the possible complications, and appropriate technique to self-inject the drug or combination of drugs advised by the urologist.

The first penile injections used papaverine. Then it was mixed with phentolamine and later with alprostadil (prostaglandin E-1). The combination of drugs works better than using them independently.

In 1995, Upjohn Laboratories had alprostadil powder approved for use as a penile injection. Caverjet comes as a dry powder, and liquid is added at the time of use. Another formula of alprostadil with an alpha-cyclo dextrin ring, called alprostadil alphadex, is manufactured by Schwarz Pharmaceuticals, and most patients can achieve a very good erection with it.

Penile Implants

Before proceeding with the implantation of a penile prosthesis, different professionals use different criteria. Urologists, understandably, are hesitant to insert a penile prosthesis when the ED is psychological. The concern is valid. Patients with psychogenic (mental/emotional) causes of ED should have a psychological or psychiatric evaluation before making the decision.

The key issue here is that the psychological reasons causing ED may be temporary. Always keep in mind that a penile prosthesis is permanent.

If we judge the effectiveness of a penile prosthesis by its ability to produce a rigid penis, the procedure can be considered a success.

The trouble is that erections per se are not always the solution for sexual interaction. Men who have poor communication skills, low sexual desire, ejaculatory problems, conflicts in the marital or personal relationship, low self-esteem, and unrealistic expectations will often go back to the doctor to express dissatisfaction with their sexual life.

Patients who suffer from psychogenic impotence may not consider the rigidity of the new penis "rigid enough." Or they may be disappointed because the penis size is smaller than before the implant.

Sometimes, a technologically induced erection is a turnoff to the sexual partner, who feels that she (or he, if the relationship is homosexual) is not capable of inducing excitement.

Because of the invasiveness involved in the implantation of a penile prosthesis, the potential complications (infections, perforations, and malfunctions), and the cost, it's preferable for most patients to consider other treatment options first.

For some men, a penile prosthesis is very gratifying, not only at a personal level, but because of the pleasure provided to the sexual partner.

Severe Dilated Cardiomyopathy, Penile Prosthesis, and "Good Sex"

Arthur was a 40-year-old man who suffered a flu-like infection. A couple of months later, he found himself with no energy, breathing difficulties, and leg swelling due to edema (fluid accumulation). The reason for all this was a very weak heart muscle with severe dilatation of the cardiac chambers (severe dilated cardiomyopathy). Arthur improved after treatment, but not enough to go back to a rather demanding job. He had also suffered from erectile failure for several years before he developed heart disease, and had had implantation of a penile prosthesis. At times, he would use the prosthesis "mostly to satisfy" his wife. That in itself gratified him a great deal. Despite his weak heart, he had a rather satisfactory sex life.

Dilated cardiomyopathies may be caused by any number of reasons, but viral infections and alcoholism are typical offenders. The outlook for these disorders varies a great deal. Sometimes there is a cure, and the heart muscle recovers its strength. Many cases follow a chronic course, and some patients require cardiac transplants.

Types of Penile Prosthesis

Penile implants can be divided into two general types: non-hydraulic and hydraulic. The former devices are also called semi-rigid prostheses, and the hydraulic types are referred to as inflatable prostheses. The prototype of the ideal candidate for a penile prosthesis is a man with a physical cause of impotence, who has tried other methods that failed, finds them unacceptable, and is considered an acceptable surgical risk.

Again, a patient who suffers from psychogenic impotence should have a psychological evaluation before consideration of penile prosthesis implantation and should consider it when sex therapy has failed and one or more sex therapists believe he could benefit from it.

The selection of the prosthesis model should be made not only by the patient but his sexual partner as well.

VIAGRA, LEVITRA, AND CIALIS

A husband to his wife after taking one of the above:

"Mary, I don't follow you. Now that I am rigid, you're asking me to be more flexible?"

The introduction of Viagra, Levitra, and Cialis is one of the most significant pharmaceutical developments of our times. They are called the PDE-5 inhibitors. Considering that erectile dysfunction (ED) has existed for as long as man has, these drugs can also be seen as one of the most formidable scientific achievements of *all* time.

Viagra was the first drug approved for oral treatment of ED by the federal Food and Drug Administration (FDA) in March of 1998. A few years later, Levitra and Cialis appeared on the market. These medications have positively influenced the lives of millions, and continue to do so at a fast pace. Their benefits are not limited to the correction of

ED. In those who respond to it—and about 70 percent of men who take them do—there are improvements in the overall quality of life, social behavior, tolerance threshold levels in the workplace, degree of patience with noisy kids at home, and understanding of other marital conflicts. They also help to deal with anxiety and depression, give hope to the lonely, generate optimism, boost self-esteem, and give a lot of people a good night's sleep, something that many did not have for a long time.

As beautiful as sexual interaction can be, historically, sex has always had its detractors. And you don't have to go that far back to find a prominent and influential doctor expressing strong negative views on sex. Sigmund Freud formulated a sex-based theory of neurosis and was himself affected by dreams of rape, incest, homosexuality, and emasculation. His ideas about sex were puritanical. He defined the sex act as degrading, believed sexual activity of any kind for pleasure, and not for procreation, was perverse, and described the perils of sexuality as "one of the most dangerous activities of the human being."

Freud wanted the conscious ego to take control of the unconscious forces in Man. Translated into sexual terms, this meant suppressing sexual impulses so that people would get rid of them and follow a life of refinement and culture. Freud was sexually inactive after age 41.

Ideas about sex vary in different social groups, and discrepancies are impressive. This happens all over the world, including the United States, of course, where multiple races, religions, and nationalities coexist. A Roman Catholic priest is ordered to be celibate. An Eastern Orthodox Catholic priest is allowed to marry and have children. Premarital virginity in women is sacred for some, but rejected and even ridiculed by others. Sex before marriage is an unavoidable necessity for many, while rejectionists see it as immoral and decadent.

The list of disagreements on sexuality goes on and on. But there is one thing, and only one, that these numerous, antagonistic, and often confrontational protagonists agree about—the desirability of an erection. They are *all* for it: Ultra-Orthodox Jews, Reformed Jews, Catholics, Evangelists, Islamic fundamentalists, Taoists, atheists, agnostics, and people of different races, nationalities, cultural backgrounds, and socioeconomic status. It isn't just a simple coincidence that 99 countries approved Viagra in less than 2 years after its approval in the United States.

Since 1998, when Viagra was released, the number of men seeking help for ED has increased impressively. What I haven't seen in my practice, however—and this is strictly a personal observation—are patients showing greater interest in discussing their sexual problems. They seem to me as secretive as those we managed in the past. What I have noticed is that patients are willing and anxious to talk about Viagra, Levitra, or Cialis.

Before Viagra, only 10 percent of men with ED in the United States consulted a doctor about it. Nowadays, many more do, although they seem to me more concerned about having an erection than delving into the possible causes of the erectile deficiency. In a way, for many men, these drugs have become the great simplifier. They bypass physical and psychological considerations, and go directly to the point. Those interested in erections now have a novel way of getting them. These medications, however, were not created to assure or guarantee success in intimate relationships.

And the explanation is simple. As important as erections are, there are other physical, psychological, emotional, and spiritual aspects that heavily influence a couple's lovemaking experience. The correction of ED is just part of a global concept, a contribution to healthy intimacy, not the ultimate, unique solution per se.

Due to a number of psychological and general health-related issues, the basic medical evaluation and work-up for ED remains as necessary and important as it was before the PDE-5 inhibitors were discovered.

Let me give an example that explains why it is important to have a medical evaluation before taking one of these drugs: Imagine a man who suffers from impotence due to undiagnosed diabetes. He gets a PDE-5 inhibitor through his "friends." The drugs "works" and he is happy about it. Two years later, diabetes is medically recognized. Conclusion: He neglected 2 years of treatment for diabetes.

Viagra, Levitra, and Cialis versus Other Treatment Options for ED

Other treatment methods for ED were described above. All of these, at one point or another, made significant contributions. And they still do, although in a more selective and limited way. Today, most of ED cases are treated with a PDE-5 inhibitor. If the drug doesn't work, it's contraindicated, or causes significant side effects, consideration is given to other treatment options. These include transurethral suppositories, intra-penile injections, surgery to correct venous leaks, vacuum pumps, and penile prostheses.

But why would anyone who can take a pill and produce an erection in 30 to 60 minutes (without adverse reactions or significant risks) want to be bothered with the side effects, risks, and inconvenience of other methods? Why put up with the occasional urethral burning of alprostadil? Why resort to a cumbersome vacuum pump that requires the penis be constricted at its base with a rubber band? Why have surgery to insert a penis prosthesis—which may at times be a great solution—when the procedure is invasive, expensive, and occasionally involves serious complications?

So, when one looks for simplicity, low risk of side effects, low complication rates, easy accessibility, effectiveness, and practicality, Viagra, Levitra, and Cialis are way ahead of the other options.

How PDE-5 Inhibitors Work

Let me first review the essential components of the penis's anatomy and the way erections normally occur.

The penis contains two chambers that run side by side along the shaft of the penis, and which are called the corpora cavernosa. The penile arteries supply blood to the corpora cavernosa through small vessels called helicine arteries. These arteries branch off into even smaller vessels called sinusoids. Smooth muscle cells surround these sinusoids. The outer edges of the corpora cavernosa are limited by the tunica albuginea. The tunica albuginea is an elastic membrane that covers the corpora cavernosa.

What produces an erection is a torrential amount of blood flow that gets into the penis during sexual excitement. The arteries carry that blood, the smooth muscles around them relax, and the penis becomes erect. Now, to maintain the erection, the blood that reached the penis, which normally exits through its veins, has to be delayed there for a while. This is assured by compression of the tunica albuginea, which is in the periphery of the corpora cavernosum. When the compression is released, the venous blood leaves the penis, and the penis "decongests" and becomes soft again.

Viagra, Levitra, and Cialis work by providing increased blood flow to the penis. Let me get just a little bit technical here and explain how these agents do that.

First, I'll describe the normal process of erection.

Hypertrophic Obstructive Cardiomyopathy: Chest Pains, Nitroglycerin, and Fainting

John was 65 and had chest pains. He fainted every time he put a nitroglycerin tablet under the tongue, and that included one occasion when he collapsed while having intercourse with his wife. His echocardiogram showed severely thickened heart muscle walls including the septum that separates both ventricles. Thick septum and left ventricular wall tend to block the exit of blood into the general circulation. Nitroglycerin aggravates this phenomenon.One of nitroglycerin effects on blood circulation is to dilate many veins. That reduces the blood return to the heart. The left ventricle is thus "half empty," which causes its walls to touch each other during cardiac contraction, blocking the exit of blood into general circulation. This happens for only a very few seconds, but it's enough to cause a fainting attack.

Nitroglycerin tablets are not recommended for patients who have severe obstructive cardiomyopathy, *even if they have angina.* Other medications can be used to control the heart muscle's contractile power, and to prevent or minimize obstruction of the left ventricular outflow tract. Severe cases at times require surgery and resection of a portion of a very thick portion of the septum.

In selected cases, a recently developed procedure has replaced surgery to reduce the thickness of the obstructing septum: ablation of the septum by injecting alcohol into it. This is done via cardiac catheterization. Serious arrhythmias, however, are sometimes seen following this "alcohol ablation of the septum" and patients require the implantation of an Intracardiac Defibrillator (ICD) that also carries a pacemaker function. I recently examined a man in his mid-thirties who had this combined treatment of septal alcohol ablation and ICD implantation, who fully recovered and played single tennis regularly and also did plenty of jogging without any cardiac symptoms.

PDE-5 Inhibitors Dosages and some peculiar characteristics

Drug	Viagra (Sildenafil) PFIZER	Levitra (Vardenafil) BAYER	Cialis (Taladafil) LILLY
Onset of action	30-60 min	30-60 min	30-60 min
Duration of effect	4 h	4h	24-36 (not always)
Dose	25-50-100 mg	2.5-5-10-20 mg	10-20 mg
Food	Fat meals reduce absorption	Fat meals reduce absorption	No food affects absorption
			May cause transient back pain

Common side effects of all the PDE-5 Inhibitors include headaches, flushing, dyspepsia (upset stomach), nasal congestion, rash, abnormal vision (blue-tinges—Viagra).

During sexual stimulation, nitric oxide (NO) is released by the parasympathetic nerves and the endothelium. Nitric oxide generates an enzyme called cGMP (cyclic guanosine monophosphate), which relaxes smooth muscle. This causes dilation of the penis arteries, increased blood flow to the penis, and the erection.

At the same time, another enzyme PDE-5 (phosphodiesterase-5) breaks down cGMP. As the level of cGMP diminishes, the smooth muscle cells contract again, and so do the arteries in the penis. The constricted arteries decrease the blood flow, the penis relaxes, and the penis becomes soft again.

Viagra, Levitra, and Cialis inhibit the production of PDE-5. This means that cGMP will not have an antagonistic factor (the PDE-5 enzyme) to face and it will be free to generate more nitric oxide (NO). This is what makes the erection possible.

Just to review:

- The smooth muscle that surrounds the arteries of the penis constricts them, limiting the blood supply. The penis is not erect.
- The smooth muscle that surrounds the arteries of the penis relaxes, increasing the blood flow. The penis becomes erect.
- The tunica albuginea compresses the veins of the penis. That reduces the exit of venous blood from the penis and the resulting congestion keeps the penis erect.

Contraindications for Using Viagra, Levitra, and Cialis

The PDE-5 inhibitors should never be taken when the patient is under treatment with any form of nitroglycerin or nitrate-derivatives, such as isosorbide, nitroglycerin capsules, transdermal nitroglycerin patches, nitroglycerin spray or inhaler, isosorbide mononitrate, or dinitrate. The combination of Viagra, Levitra, or Cialis with these drugs may cause a precipitous and dangerous lowering of the blood pressure.

Hypotensive states (low blood pressure) may be caused by medications prescribed for prostatic enlargement (terazosin, doxazosin), excessive use of diuretics (water pills); severe anemia; a condition called "orthostatic hypotension," which causes marked blood pressure reductions on standing up; severe aortic valvular stenosis (calcified aortic valve), important cardiac rhythm disturbances, and/or dehydration.

Take this example: A fit 72-year-old man plays tennis, doesn't drink fluids, and perspires profusely during the game. His blood pressure falls to 90/60. His usual blood pressure is 140/80. He feels weak, but well otherwise. He goes home, intending to have sex with his wife. He takes any of the PDE-5 inhibitors, his blood pressure falls even further, down to 60/0, and he faints.

Viagra, Levitra, or Cialis need to be prescribed by a physician who knows your medical and cardiovascular history and is familiar with your blood pressure fluctuations—or the possibility that such fluctuations might occur.

Some Cautionary Notes

If you take any of the PDE-5 inhibitors, get involved in lovemaking, and then develop anginal discomfort, stop sexual activity and relax. If the chest discomfort is mild and lasts for 2 to 3 minutes, continue to rest and do not resume any kind of sexual effort the same night. If the pain is more severe and lasts longer than usual, call 911 or your physician. Never put a nitroglycerin tablet under the tongue.

If a rescue team assists you at home, immediately tell them that you took Viagra, Levitra, or Cialis, so you will not be given a nitroglycerin preparation. These drugs are very safe, but, like any other medications, you must use them the way you are supposed to. If you take a drug at the wrong time and under the wrong conditions, you may have a reaction. It won't be the medication's fault, but the misguided way it was used.

Drugs Well Tolerated with Viagra, Levitra, and Cialis

- Alcohol (must avoid excessive consumption or intoxicating levels. A significant blood pressure drop might be hazardous.)

- Antacids
- Antidepressants
- Antidiabetic drugs
- Antihypertensives
- Aspirin
- Lipid-lowering medications
- Warfarin

Special Precautions

- Never take Viagra, Levitra, or Cialis when you are taking nitro-glycerin or nitrate-derivatives. Consult your physician about any medical condition where any of these drugs should be temporarily or permanently avoided. (See Contraindications on page 202.)
- Avoid these drugs if you have had any serious cardiovascular event in the past 6 months (myocardial infarction, stroke, life-threatening arrhythmia, recent heart failure, and unstable angina), until your doctor suggests when to resume them. Do not take them if you have uncontrolled hypertension (resting blood pressure greater than 170/110) or hypotension (resting blood pressure 90/60 or lower).
- If you have retinitis pigmentosa, consult an ophthalmologist before using PDE-5 inhibitors.
- If you experience sudden decrease or loss of vision while taking any of the PDE-5 inhibitors, see an ophthalmologist immediately.
- If you develop a painful erection that persists longer than 4 hours, go to an emergency room and get examined by a urologist. This condition requires immediate medical attention.

- If you are taking protease inhibitors, such as those used to treat HIV, your doctor may recommend a low dose of the PDE-5 inhibitor, and you may be advised NOT to repeat it for 48 hours.
- If you are older than age 65, or have serious liver or kidney disease, your doctor may start you at the lowest possible dose of any of the PDE-5 inhibitors.
- If you have a curved penis (Peronie's disease), do not take Viagra, Levitra, or Cialis without consulting a urologist first. Surgical correction of this condition is usually indicated prior to taking any of these drugs.

Successful Treatment of ED in the Presence of Other Medical Conditions

A remarkable therapeutic effect of the PDE-5 inhibitors is that they can be successful in treating ED whatever the cause, including:

- Atherosclerosis
- Depression
- Diabetes
- Psychological conflicts
- Radical prostatectomy
- Spinal cord injuries

The Reported Association between Viagra and Fatalities

From March of 1998, when Viagra was introduced, until mid-November of 1998, approximately 6 million prescriptions of Viagra were written. At the same time, the FDA reported 130 deaths. Since most of these patients suffered from cardiovascular disease, smoking, obesity, hypertension, and diabetes, it is very difficult to link these fatalities to Viagra. There is a possibility that some of these deaths might have been related to the fact that some patients combined the drug with nitrates.

Many men who *die daily* from cardiovascular disease are not taking Viagra, Levitra, Cialis, or having sexual activity.

These drugs have an extraordinary safety record, which has been documented in clinical trials and corroborated by similar results in millions of individuals.

A Revolution

PDE-5 inhibitors have indeed caused a revolution, if we define "revolution" as the deployment of innovative technology that successfully deals with one of the most distressing afflictions suffered by men for countless centuries. And when you think about it, and see that so many individuals change the course of their lives and become happier and more productive because of a tiny pill, you just can't help being moved by the achievement.

Revolutions in medicine are not new. The discovery of penicillin was revolutionary, and this marvelous drug saved millions, but it still causes 400 deaths from allergic reactions in the United States every year. Blood transfusions were also revolutionary, and we are grateful for the gift of life they give to so many, but they have claimed numerous victims because of the co-transmission of hepatitis, AIDS, and other contaminants. Prosthetic cardiac valves revolutionized the treatment of valvular heart disease, but there were mechanical failures that took decades to correct, and many people paid their dues for those defects.

The beauty of the PDE-5 inhibitors revolution is that these drugs are usually effective *and* safe.

From the above discussion and the various alternatives available to deal with ED, you may have the impression that the selection of an appropriate therapy is a complicated issue. Well, really, it is not. The basic issue here is to rely on professionals who are sensitive to your problem and have the motivation and expertise to show that little, and yet, hopeful light, that flushes at the end of the tunnel

CONCLUSION

The treatment options for ED are:

1. Oral medications (Viagra, Levitra, Cialis)
2. Local treatments:
      Intra-penile injections (intracorporeal injections)
      Intra-urethral suppositories
3. Surgical treatments:
      Penile prosthesis
      Revascularization

I want to close this chapter mentioning the observations of two eminent American psychotherapists who have extensive research and clinical experience in the field of sex therapy. Dr. Sandra R. Leiblum and Dr. Raymond C. Cohen have identified the three most frequently encountered couple's conflicts in cases of ED *(Principles and Practice of Sex Therapy-Guilford, 3rd Edition)*. These are: "Status and dominance issues, intimacy and trust, and loss of sexual attraction."

Status and dominance issues arise when the balance of power in a relationship is shifted, either because of external factors such as loss of a job and unemployment or because of internal factors such as depression and loss of self-esteem. "Intimacy and trust difficulties may occur when either partner engages in an extramarital affair, undertakes a new career, or gives birth to a child. Loss of sexual attraction may be associated with weight gain, medical illnesses or surgery, and abuse of drugs or alcohol."

From the above discussion and the various alternatives available to deal with ED, you may have the impression that the selection of appropriate therapy is a complicated issue. Well, really, it is not. The basic issue here is to rely on professionals who are sensitive to your problem and have the motivation and expertise to show you that little, and yet, hopeful light that flashes at the end of the tunnel.

Chapter 16

Exercise, the Heart, and Sex

The heart's favorite sport is moderation.

The effects of exercise on the heart have recently been the focus of considerable interest. One of the reasons for this has been the explosive enthusiasm that many people developed for strenuous exercise—thinking that it can prevent or cure heart disease. There's no argument about the fact that regular physical exercise has a salutary effect on the cardiovascular system. What must be kept in mind, however, is that exercise is not a safe proposition at all times and not for everybody.

For patients who have coronary artery disease—regardless of whether they have or haven't had a myocardial infarction, balloon angioplasty, or coronary bypass surgery—exercise is very important. Exercise is also desirable for people who don't have cardiovascular disease, but do want to have excellent physical conditioning.

There is also an important connection between exercise, cardiovascular health, and sexuality. Regular exercise increases stamina, flexibility, and breathing capacity. The implications for a better sex life are obvious, not only from the physical standpoint but in terms of self-confidence and lack of fear regarding the body's capabilities.

Sexual activity is a form of exercise. For more information on energy expenditure and physical demands of sexual activity, please see Chapter 14.

Physical exercise can be a gratifying experience when properly handled, but improperly managed, it can be troublesome. You should know the type of exercise you're medically allowed to have, how much of it you should do, and be aware of its limitations.

STATIC VERSUS DYNAMIC EXERCISE

To understand the concept of "static versus dynamic exercise," remember this: you have a pump (the heart) and an arterial system throughout the body. Exercise changes both—in different ways—depending upon the type of exercise you do.

Static (or isometric) exercise, such as weightlifting, minimally increases the ejection of blood from the heart, and causes widespread arterial vasoconstriction. This means that the muscles in action may actually receive less blood than they usually do. This type of exercise also uses small groups of muscles.

Because of the vasoconstriction, blood pressure increases. That in turn limits the ejection of blood by the heart pump, so blood volume is actually lower than normal. The lower volume of blood ejected by the heart and the vasoconstriction in the arterial vessels cause a decrease in the amount of oxygen delivered to tissues. Thus, static exercise is also called anaerobic exercise.

Dynamic (or isotonic) exercise, such as walking and jogging, increases the volume of blood ejected by the heart (called stroke volume) and causes arterial vasodilatation. The greater volume of blood ejected and the dilatation of arteries increase blood flow to all body organs and tissues, and thus more oxygen is delivered as well. This kind of exercise also uses large groups of muscles. Dynamic exercise is also called aerobic exercise.

The cardiovascular benefits of exercise mostly result from aerobic (dynamic) physical activity.

CARDIOVASCULAR CONDITIONING

Cardiovascular conditioning may be viewed as an ongoing adaptation of the cardiovascular system reached by consistent, progressive exercise. Heart rate and blood pressure tend to drop as physical conditioning improves. The increase in heart rate observed during exercise is responsible for the larger output of blood from the cardiac chambers.

Exercise dilates coronary arteries, and this applies to the large coronary vessels as much as to microcirculation—that is, the heart's tiniest branches. This represents an adaptation of the coronary circulation, which provides increased blood supply when the heart muscle requires it.

DAILY WORKOUT ROUTINES

What follows are general concepts that will help you to understand how exercise planning works.

Intensity of Exercise

Physical fitness and good physical and cardiovascular conditioning are usually achieved when a person exercises regularly between 50 percent and 80 percent of his or her functional capacity. "Functional capacity" is another way of saying "maximum heart rate." Your optimal, maximum heart rate can be grossly estimated by subtracting your age from 220. For example, if you are 50 years of age, your maximum heart rate is 220 minus 50 or 170 beats per minute.

Now, if you exercise at a rate of 60 percent your functional capacity (or maximum heart rate), that means you are exercising at 60 percent of 170 beats per minute—or 102 beats per minute.

If you exercise at a rate of 80 percent of your functional capacity (maximum heart rate), that means you are exercising at 80 percent of 170 beats per minute—or 136 beats per minute.

Frequency of Exercise

Three times a week is the minimum exercise required to achieve some degree of physical conditioning. Five to seven times a week provides better results, but you have to be careful to avoid sprains, injuries, or doing more exercise than advised by your physician. Each patient, and in fact, each person, needs an individualized approach. Exercise programs thus have to be designed individually.

Place of Exercise

Some people prefer walking exercises in the street. Others are happy at the gym or at home with their own equipment. Some need a personal trainer. Without this kind of support, they can't function well. Personal taste and other factors, including economics, influence this decision.

Physical activities that promote good cardiovascular conditioning include jogging, walking, bicycling, swimming, sports, calisthenics, yoga, and rowing, to name just some.

Vigorous housework and gardening are helpful, too.

When using the treadmill, you can determine the progress you have achieved by measuring your workout performance with numbers. One week you may walk at 2.8 miles per hour for 30 minutes. Next week you can increase the speed to 3.1 miles per hour, and so on. Buying a treadmill isn't too expensive these days.

If you suffer from neck or low back pains, consult an orthopedic doctor before doing treadmill exercises. Sometimes, these pains can become aggravated.

Light weights for exercising arms, shoulders, chest, and back should not be forgotten during your workouts, as they help to preserve muscular tone and strength.

Duration of Exercise

With your doctor's approval, aim to exercise from 30 to 60 minutes daily, if possible, at your target heart rate (50 percent to 80 percent of your maximum heart rate). If you get bored with prolonged sessions, or get tired, try two shorter sessions a day. Go gradually. Don't push yourself. Note: Before you increase your level (intensity) of physical exercise, first increase its duration (length).

Respect the Three Stages of an Exercise Session

Warm-up phase: Stretch the muscles of the areas you intend to use. (Before using the treadmill, for example, do some stretching of leg muscles for 10 minutes before working out. This will help avoid unnecessary sprains.)

Exercise phase: Plan on doing 30 to 60 minutes of exercise.

Cool-down phase: This is a gradual reduction of the level of exercise. Some individuals feel lightheaded when they abruptly end the exercise. Here's why: During exercise, the venous return to the heart increases because the muscles (mostly the lower extremities) squeeze the veins and contribute to the filling of the cardiac chambers. If exercise is stopped abruptly, the squeezing stops and venous return to the heart is decreased. This results in decreased ejection of blood from the heart, the brain then receives less blood than it's used to, and this in turn causes lightheadedness.

Don't mix food or alcohol with exercise!

When you eat a meal, the blood supply to the digestive system increases, and so does the heart's work. Trying to exercise right after eating puts an unnecessary burden on the heart. Wait several hours after a meal, preferably 3 to 4, before you exercise. Alcohol increases the chances of having cardiac arrhythmias.

EVALUATION OF A CARDIAC PATIENT PRIOR TO EXERCISE

Cardiac patients need an evaluation of their cardiac status before they engage in physical exercise. Various types of stress tests are available for this purpose. The most basic is the regular treadmill stress test. This is done by just walking on the treadmill without being injected nuclear material. Others require it.

Contraindications to Exercise Stress Testing

An exercise stress test must not be done when the patient has any of the following conditions:

- Acute myocardial infarction
- Large abdominal aortic aneurysm (AAA)
- Severe aortic valvular stenosis (tight narrowing of the aortic valve)
- Severe hypertension (for example: 180/110)
- Severe hypertrophic obstructive cardiomyopathy (marked thickening of portions of the cardiac muscle that interfere with the ejection of blood into the general circulation)
- Severe low serum potassium
- Severe mental or physical impairment that limits a person's capacity to exercise adequately
- Uncontrolled rapid heart rates (tachycardia), or very slow heart rates (bradycardia)

❤ Unstable angina (increase in the frequency and severity of chest discomfort or pain resulting from blockages of coronary arteries)

Exercise and Cardiovascular Death in the General Population

The annual incidence of sudden death in individuals under the age of thirty is between two and seven deaths per 100,000, of which 8 percent are exercise-related. In persons over age 30, the incidence of sudden death is between 50 and 60 deaths per 100,000, of which approximately 2 to 3 percent occur during exercise. Most of these deaths occur in those with unrecognized or "silent" heart disease. Among young people, the rate of sudden death due to coronary heart disease is about 5 percent. The remaining deaths are due to a number of other heart conditions; for example, arrhythmias and cardiomyopathies. In older populations, coronary involvement accounts for about ⅔ of sudden cardiac death cases.

Overall, the prevailing scientific view is that for the majority of the population, including select patients with coronary artery disease, carefully prescribed physical conditioning is safe and may benefit the individual by helping strengthen the cardiovascular system, and/or by preventing or postponing the onset of coronary artery disease.

Chapter 17

Nutrition and Your Heart

PHYSICIAN: "Johnny, you have to believe this. We are what we eat."

PATIENT: "Is that so? Really? Doctor, please, GIVE ME A DIET RIGHT
AWAY!"

If you are an average American, or a foreigner who has been living in the United States for a number of years, chances are that
you've been consuming unhealthy foods for a long time; conceiv-
ably, since you were born.

I don't have to go too far to find an example. Look at me. I was
raised in Argentina. Its beautiful prairies, called *Las Pampas,* produced
herds of cattle, and food was plentiful. Parents wanted their children
to be healthy and strong. So, I was brought up in a culture of meat,
eggs, and dairy products. And ice creams, cakes, and pastries.
Delicious pastries. Unforgettable pastries. Unhealthy pastries.

How did I survive this repetitive assault on my body cells and
blood lipids, and so far, not had heart trouble? I don't know. I guess
I was lucky. Very lucky, indeed. But I've also changed. I eat differently these days, and, I should add, much better. I am careful about both
the quantity and quality of the foods I consume.

Many authorities agree on the following: The typical American
(Western) diet, based on meat, dairy products, and simple carbohy-

drates (beef, chicken, pork, eggs, cheese, butter, margarine, hydrogenated oils, chocolate, ice cream, doughnuts, cakes, pastries, cookies), with an abundance of white flower and white sugar, causes disturbances in blood lipids that lead to atherosclerosis. Obesity and a sedentary lifestyle are closely associated with poor eating habits, and are also major contributors. If diabetes, stress, and smoking join the club, risks are not only added, but multiplied.

Basic knowledge of nutrition is essential for protection of your heart and sexual functioning. Sexual dysfunctions often result from cardiovascular disease induced by bad eating habits. If you load your arteries with fatty deposits—and have a stroke, heart attack, or blockages of the arteries that supply blood to the genitals—your sexual performance will be in jeopardy.

VEGAN VERSUS BURGERS: THE PROS AND CONS OF DIETS FOR PATIENTS WITH OBESITY AND CORONARY ARTERY DISEASE

Numerous diets are promoted to deal with obesity. Just take a visit to the diet book section of a major bookstore. You'll be amazed at the number of publications that promote drastically different weight-reducing programs. At one point, you may feel you could lose weight by doing or eating almost anything. And, in an almost funny twist of biological expediency, that statement contains an element of truth.

It's a fact that you can lose weight by focusing only on meat derivatives, or by displaying new vegetarian credentials. I've seen enough of both methods to tell you that they frequently work. The sticky point is not what diet makes you lose weight, but rather, what the effects are of such a diet on your future health. If you suffer from coronary artery disease, you have to be especially careful.

So, losing weight is important, but what happens to you in the process deserves attention and raises justified concerns. There are safe and unsafe ways to lose weight. If you decide to lose weight fast by unsafe means, I can guarantee that there is a price to be paid. It's essential to normalize your weight, but you *must* use a method that will not hurt you.

Opposing dietary and weight-loss views are held by vegans (vegetarians who consume no meat, dairy products, or eggs) and by advocates of high-protein, high-fat, low-carbohydrate diets.

In everyday practice, however, I see patients offering great resistance to vegetarian rules and regulations. I struggle to modify my patients' eating habits and lifestyles, and I consider myself a medical Olympic champion when I convince one of them that eating French fries and double cheeseburgers is not in his or her best interest. As far as the famous Atkins diet goes (high protein, high fat, low carbohydrates), which typically wakes you up with a breakfast that includes a cheese and broccoli omelet with bacon and/or sausage, I do not recommend it. Sprinkling saturated fats into circulatory systems and risking the formation or cracking of atherosclerotic plaques is a frightening prospect. I do not support this diet, even in people without cardiovascular disease. Many organizations also oppose high-protein, high-fat, and low-carbohydrate diets, including the American Heart Association, the American Cancer Society, the World Health Organization, the American Dietetic Association, and the Surgeon General of the United States.

There is another method for reversal of coronary artery disease. It is advocated by K. Lance Gould, M.D., Professor and Founding Director of the Weatherhead PET Imaging Center for Preventing and Reversing Heart Disease. Dr. Gould also served as Director of Cardiology at the University of Texas Medical School in Houston. He has extensive clinical and research experience on reversal therapy for coronary artery disease.

PRINCIPLES OF REVERSAL (ALSO CALLED REGRESSION) THERAPY

Some atherosclerotic plaques remain flat and intact for the rest of a person's life, while others grow to block the lumen of arteries. These plaques can be localized or involve a longer segment of the artery.

A main objective of reversal treatment is to significantly reduce blood cholesterol levels. This both reduces deposits of LDL cholesterol particles on the arterial wall and facilitates their removal. The fibrous cap flattens and tends to adhere to the wall of the coronary artery. Removal of lipid particles from the plaque reduces the risk of plaque rupture.

HDL particles are in charge of removing LDL particles from the arterial wall. This job is best done when HDL cholesterol levels are high. HDL particles remove and transport LDL cholesterol to the liver, which does what it can to dispose of them.

Although the reduction in plaque size with successful reversal therapy is not great—about 8 percent after 4 to 5 years, as measured by computer-analyzed quantitative angiograms—the overall clinical response is significant. Blood flow to the heart muscle substantially increases, as demonstrated by PET cardiac scans.

This is followed by a dramatic improvement in cardiac disease symptoms and outcomes. There is a significant reduction of unstable angina, myocardial infarctions, strokes, and death, and a decrease in the need for balloon angioplasty, stents, and coronary bypass surgery.

THE EXTRAORDINARY IMPORTANCE OF SIGNIFICANT BLOOD LIPIDS REDUCTION

Reversal treatment does not aim for normal cholesterol levels. The target numbers we are going to mention below are lower than those defined by the American Heart Association as normal. Many patients involved with this form of therapy often improve quickly, and see a reduction in the frequency and severity of chest pains, shortness of breath, and fatigue in a few weeks.

Target Serum Lipids Levels for Partial Regression of Atherosclerosis

- Total cholesterol: Below 140 mg/dl
- LDL cholesterol: Below 70 mg/dl
- HDL cholesterol: Over 50 mg/dl for men and over 55 mg/dl for women
- Triglycerides: Below 130 mg/dl

Reversal or regressive therapy is appropriate for people who have coronary artery disease or for those who are at great risk for developing it. The implementation of this therapy requires a radical change in lifestyle and a permanent commitment. The method is very good—and it's for real—but it demands performance, discipline, and consistency. It is not to be taken casually. Keep this in mind: Casual approaches yield casual results.

The basic components of reversal therapy are listed below.

- Lower LDL cholesterol as much as possible.
- Raise HDL cholesterol as much as possible.
- Achieve target cholesterol levels through diet and medications when necessary. Complement cholesterol treatment, when feasible, by eliminating other cardiovascular risk factors.
- Follow a program of regular exercise that is first approved by your doctor, with specific instructions on how much you may exercise per day or per week.
- Normalize weight.
- Control hypertension. See Appendix B.

- Control diabetes. Target A1C glycohemoglobin levels should be less than 6 percent.
- Control stress. Read pertinent literature; try yoga and/meditation; seek psychological or psychiatric counseling; confront stress in your own unique way, including doing some serious soul-searching.
- Smoking cessation. If you still have a cigarette ready for ignition, you have to work on that deficiency *fast*.

DIETARY GUIDELINES FOR REVERSAL THERAPY

Following is a summary of Dr. K. Lance Gould's food guidelines. Remember, the general diet principle here is: low carbohydrates, very low fats, and adequate protein

- Eat no fat or very low fat foods. Eliminate margarine, oils, butter, and all identifiable fat. Any food with more than 1 to 2 grams of fat per serving should be avoided.
- Get adequate protein from nonfat sources, particularly nonfat dairy products, but also from occasional servings of fish, turkey, chicken breast, yolk-free eggs, and veggie burgers.
- Reduce or eliminate large volume carbohydrate sources, such as rice, bread, potatoes, pasta, pastries, sweets, fruit juice, and bananas, in order to reach ideal weight, reduce triglycerides, and increase HDL levels. Substitute protein, vegetables, and up to three fruits per day for the fats and carbohydrates eliminated from diet. After reaching lean body mass, increase these carbohydrates in amounts sufficient to maintain weight. Fill up on large amounts of vegetables—raw, steamed, or stir-fried without oil.
- Never get too hungry. Snack often if needed. If hungry, eat

large amounts of only the right foods, principally vegetables and nonfat protein with some fruit. Add rice, bread, potatoes, and pasta in modest amounts only when ideal weight is reached.

- Do the right food shopping. Meal preparation will be simpler and quicker.
- Read labels on food products for fat, carbohydrate, and protein content.
- Once a month, eat a favorite food that is not part of the new diet.
- Develop an upbeat attitude. Think of low-fat and low–carbohydrate foods in a positive way.

To summarize: Vegetables represent the largest volume of food in this diet, followed by protein. Following protein, fruits are added, with are more allowed for lean people. The next level of food consumption is bulk carbohydrates like bread, pasta, rice, potatoes, pastries, and sweets. These foods must be consumed in very limited quantities to achieve lean body weight. At the end of the food options lies fat, which should be the smallest component of one's diet.

Dr. Gould's guidelines stress an optimal food plan to achieve lean body weight by both carbohydrate and fat reduction, with adequate protein from nonfat, low-carbohydrate sources, and volumes of vegetables for fiber and phyto–nutrients. These protein sources include nonfat dairy products, such as nonfat yogurt, nonfat cheese, skim milk, nonfat cottage cheese, egg whites, veggie burgers, or soy protein, supplemented with some breast of turkey or chicken, fish, or buffalo venison. Cholesterol intake should be limited to between 60 and 80 mg a day, and fat to 10 percent of total daily calories.

The typical American diet contains 40 to 50 percent fat (mostly saturated) and 400 to 500 mg cholesterol per day. The reversal diet reduces daily fat consumption to 10 percent or less of mostly monounsaturated and polyunsaturated fats. Carbohydrate intake varies according to weight. Lean body mass is the objective. During the weight-reducing program, carbohydrates are restricted. Later, they can be added to the diet if the added amount does not cause weight gain.

It is acceptable to eat more than 60 to 80 grams of protein per day. For those who need increased protein intake to feel more satisfied, protein can be increased to 100 to 150 grams a day, but in such cases, fat should not be higher than 15 to 20 grams a day.

Now, to be candid, many patients do not easily accept restricted diets. People like to eat, and for many individuals, food restrictions represent the ultimate sacrifice. Some will tell you that it would be easier for them to become president of the United States than to give up their heavy-duty New York sirloin steaks, potatoes loaded with sour cream, and voluminous ice cream sundaes, including the decorative single cherry on top.

Whatever diet you choose, you must be convinced that it is going to work for you, not against you. And if it doesn't make you happy, it at least shouldn't make you miserable, either. You need to reach a compromise, a kind of negotiated settlement between your psyche and your gastric juices. In other words, you need to trade many gastronomic pleasures for a safer cardiovascular future.

During the initial stages of this new diet, you may not always be able to resist temptation. If you yield to it, don't feel remorseful and guilty about it. Do better next time, and keep on trying until you get it right. Train yourself to develop stronger willpower. If you decide to do some cheating occasionally (I'm only referring to food), do it in an organized way: Select one day a month and eat something you miss. Then go right back to your diet and the discipline you need to achieve regression of your coronary artery disease. In the end, if you feel that this new restricted diet is giving you nothing but suffering and deprivation, don't forget what the alternatives are: recurrent chest pains, myocardial infarctions, hospitalizations, physical, psychological, social and relationship problems, repeated balloon angioplasties, coronary bypass surgeries, *and* sexual limitations.

Conclusion

The human's greatest hope is to have a second chance.

In pursuing your goals and trying to assimilate new ideas and put them into practice, more often than not you will make mistakes. And when you plan something as difficult as a radical change in lifestyle—which is most likely what you need—you must be ready to face "performance errors" and deal with them. This, however, should not distract you from your main objective or deter you from having constructive, positive attitudes.

THE INEVITABLE AND THE AVOIDABLE

Some cardiac disorders are inevitable: congenital heart disease, weakness of the heart muscle resulting from a viral infection, or a heart that becomes dilated and flabby after delivery, and no one knows why. And so many others. Nevertheless, it is a fact that the majority of patients suffering from cardiovascular disease have inflicted it on themselves. Basic lifestyles rules are ignored, and people often act as if they were assaulting their own bodies with smoking, excessive alcohol, hot dogs, hamburgers (and please, don't forget the cheese on top), French fries floating in toxic oil, cakes, cookies, ice cream sundaes, stress, depression, conflicts at work and at home, poor control of cholesterol, diabetes, hypertension, and insufficient physical exercise.

What's the origin of such neglect? There are many reasons: lack of awareness, insufficient education, personality disorders, psychological dysfunctions of various kinds, immaturity, denial, stubbornness, laziness, lack of will power. Choose anyone you want. It'll do it.

The correction of human dysfunctional behavior is what's really needed. But let's face it: Psychologists have a most difficult time trying to make a difference. You must recognize that succeeding in changing a lifestyle radically is not an easy proposition. The vast majority of patients, at least the patients I see in my daily practice, cannot do it. A selective minority are totally successful, another minority are notoriously unsuccessful, but the majority fall into an intermediate category: they try corrective actions, but they struggle between what they do and what they are supposed to do. They may do better. But doing better does not mean *doing well.* Reducing cholesterol levels from 260 to 230 is a little better, but is definitely not good; the same holds true for smoking 20 cigarettes a day instead of 40; going from 85 pounds overweight to 55 pounds overweight, and increasing physical exercise from doing nothing to walking fast for 15 minutes, once a week.

All these improvements are certainly preferable to no improvements at all, but cardiovascular risks remain disturbingly high. And so do risks of sexual dysfunction and life disruption.

Sexual performance and cardiovascular risk factors go hand in hand. Poor diets and obesity contribute to diabetes, and many diabetic patients suffer from sexual dysfunction. Uncontrolled hypertension does the same. Smokers who have significant chronic lung disease are fatigued and short of breath, and so are those who have had a big chunk of lung tissue removed because of tobacco-induced cancer. Those who have high cholesterol blood levels—and have heart attacks or strokes as a result—also face temporary or permanent disruption of their sexual capabilities. The list of cardiovascular risk factors that can affect sexual functioning (actually, all of them do), can be reviewed in Appendix B.

TRYING FOR A SOLUTION

Always keep in mind that prevention is preferable to treatment. The best way to solve a problem is never to have it. But if you already have a problem, these are the steps I suggest you follow.

1. Analysis: Identification of problems
2. Action: Execution of a plan

Please, see the analysis sheet below. Circle the items that represent your problems. This is followed by the medical assessment of the identified problems.

ACTION

This is the final step in the implementation of radical lifestyle changes. To be effective, conception, planning, and execution of corrective methods need to be consistent, thoughtful, and methodical.

Evaluate the contribution (percentage-wise) of the following problems (cardiac, medical, psychological, and so on) to your sexual dysfunction. Your physician's assistance is essential. It is very important to identify the cause (or causes) of the sexual dysfunction as much as possible. For instance, a male suffering from diabetes may believe that this disease is causing his erectile failure, but this may not be necessarily the case. He may be having marital conflicts or stress due to other reasons that are truly responsible for his poor erections. A woman may blame menopause for her orgasmic dysfunction, but the real reason may be a deceptive intimate relationship, or a side effect from an antidepressant.

227

	Example	YOU
Coronary artery disease	10%	___
Medical illnesses	5%	___
Habits (smoking, drinking, recreational drugs, etc.)	0%	___
Psychological status	5%	___
Drugs (medications), prescribed and/or over-the-counter	10%	___
Family—social—economic conditions	0%	___
Poor quality of the relationship	70%	___

Once you have analyzed the possible causes of the sexual dysfunction, you will be able to approach their tentative solutions in a specific manner. Please, note in the above example the great contribution of poor quality of the relationship to the sexual dysfunction: 70 percent. The conclusion is clear: drugs or methods to deal with erectile failure will not produce results. What is needed is an in-depth evaluation of the marital relationship which is best done by a psychotherapist.

Well, the time has come to say "So long." So, let me share with you some thoughts. We all wish to be happy. That is our great desire and design. To achieve happiness, we need to enjoy good mental and physical health. Lots of people lack the natural talent to take good care of themselves. But the knowledge to be physically, mentally, and emotionally healthy can be acquired.

Those interested in learning more about heart attacks, cardiovascular risk factors, and some tips on commonly used cardiac drugs are referred

Analysis Sheet

Cardiovascular Disease	Medical Illnesses	Habits	Drugs
Coronary artery disease	Diabetes	Smoking	Beta-blocker
Hypertension	Emphysema	Alcohol	Digitalis
Valvular heart disease	Kidney failure	Marijuana	Nitrates
Cardiomyopathy	Blood disorder	Cocaine	Diuretic
Pericarditis	Thyroid gland disease	Sedentary lifestyle	Steroids
Arrhythmia	Liver disease		Ace-Inhibitors
Stroke	Severe arthritis	Chemotherapy	
Aortic aneurysm	Blood lipids		OTC (*)
Carotid artery blockage	Cancer		
Legs arterial obstructions	Neurological disorder		
Congenital heart disease	Gastrointestinal disease		
Renal artery blockage	Hormonal disorder		
Other	Other		

to the Appendixes. In the main section of the book, I mostly focused on subjects that relate more closely to the heart and sex. I'd like to remind you that the information we provide in the Appendixes is valuable not only for prevention and treatment of cardiovascular disease but for the preservation of your sexual functioning as well. Good sexual performance and good cardiovascular health are inseparable companions.

There is currently a wealth of information available to those who want to learn at all educational levels. You have access to history books, literature, humor, fishing, cooking, psychology books, all kinds of books,

Sexual Performance

Non-existent
Very poor
Poor

Acceptable
Satisfactory
Very Satisfactory

Psychological Status

Anxiety Depression
Bipolar disorder
OCD (**)

Panic attacks
PTSD (***)
Other

Quality of the Relationship

Excellent
Very good
Good

Fair
Poor
Unacceptable
Other

Family-Social-Economic conditions

Financial hardship
Stressful job
Unemployment
Dangerous Neighborhood

Intrusive relatives
Religious conflicts
Other

(*) OTC: Over the counter medications
(**) OCD: Obsessive-compulsive disorder
(***) PTSD: Post-traumatic stress disorder

including sex books, sex movies, sex videos, sex shops. All you have to do is to ring the bell of your imagination and rub the magic lamp. When the genie comes out of it and is ready to grant you anything you want, just ask him to gift you with a positive and cheerful attitude when dealing with the problems of the present, and the uncertainties of the future.

I wish you my best.

—*Ed Chapunoff*

Appendix A

Anatomy of a Heart Attack

DISCLAIMER

What you will find in the following appendices is not meant to replace or even to supplement information given to you by your doctor. If you are suffering from any sort of heart illness, I urge you to go to the Resource section of this text and contact the relevant institution, and read as much as you can find on your illness. The following information is meant to clarify and explain some of the terms used previously in the text, and to be only the beginning of your search for information.

THE ENDOTHELIUM

The endothelium can be the source of disease and carries great destructive potential. It is the inner lining of the arteries that comprise your entire vascular tree—all the arteries in your body. It is made up of a single layer of endothelial cells and is the most extensive tissue in the body.

The circulating blood is in direct contact with endothelial cells. When these are intact, blood flows smoothly. When the endothelial cells become damaged, (by high levels of cholesterol, hypertension, smoking, diabetes, etc.), LDL or "bad cholesterol" particles invade the endothelial layer and contribute to the formation of the atherosclerotic plaque. If, for some reason, the plaque suffers a crack, substances circulating in the blood interact with those released by the disrupted plaque and produce a clot. If the clot is small, it will partially obstruct the artery and the patient may experience chest pains that are more prolonged and severe than usual. If the clot is large enough to block the artery completely, the heart muscle is acutely deprived of blood supply and the acute myocardial infarction ensues.

Atherosclerotic plaques can cause varying degrees of arterial obstruction. A 50 percent or less reduction of the arterial lumen (lumen is the space inside the artery where the blood circulates) is not considered a significant blockage because the blood flow through the narrowed area is not affected. Lesions that block 75 percent or more of the artery are significant because the blood flow is reduced. Soft, mildly obstructive lesions are also capable of causing acute myocardial infarctions because they break easily. Hard, calcified plaques are less vulnerable, and do not crack so easily.

THE DIFFERENCE BETWEEN MYOCARDIAL ISCHEMIA AND MYOCARDIAL INFARCTION

The myocardium is a muscular pump that propels blood into the circulation. The heart is no ordinary pump: In seventy-five years, it contracts 3.26 billion times, and in that period, it ejects 57.5 million gallons of blood. The "fuel" the myocardium needs to do its work is the blood provided by three major coronary arteries and their branches.

The coronary arteries arise from the aorta. The blood carries red cells transporting oxygen to the heart tissue. Insufficient delivery of oxygen adversely affects the heart muscle. When this is not associated with heart muscle damage the condition is called ischemia (pronounced IS-KEE-MIA). When there is cardiac muscle damage, it's called a myocardial infarction.

When there is prolonged and complete interruption of blood supply to the cardiac muscle for over 15 to 20 minutes, a myocardial infarction takes place. In other words, ischemia is reversible deficiency of blood supply. Reversible means that the heart muscle will regain its vitality if some form of treatment (or nature itself) allows fresh blood to reach the compromised area. This fresh blood comes from the dissolution of small clots in the coronary artery due either to:

- ♥ the patient's natural clot-dissolving mechanisms
- ♥ the presence of collateral circulation that diverts blood to the suffering area from a neighboring area
- ♥ prompt and effective medical treatment that includes intravenous administration of a clot-dissolving drug
- ♥ balloon angioplasty
- ♥ coronary bypass surgery
- ♥ or any of the preceding in combination.

A myocardial infarction is permanent damage of the cardiac muscle produced by sudden interruption of the blood supply. Cardiac cells that had been nourished by the now affected coronary artery die. Once that happens, the muscle damage is irreversible and a scar replaces what used to be healthy heart muscle. Since scars do not contract actively as the rest of the cardiac muscle does, they represent useless tissue. When the damaged area is small, future cardiac function may not be affected. Sizable myocardial infarctions, however, reduce the heart's contractile power and may lead to arrhythmias and heart failure.

It is very desirable to discover the presence of ischemia before it progresses to an infarction. If a myocardial infarction is on its way, we want it to be as small as possible, and if it has already occurred, we want to do everything possible to prevent a recurrence.

It's likely that you may be totally unaware of the existence of both ischemia and infarction. There are multiple episodes of ischemia that produce no symptoms, that happens during the day or night. In fact, such ischemic episodes may occur during the sleep (and so do myocardial infarctions). When ischemia causes chest pains, chest discomfort, or other symptoms, the patient is symptomatic.

UNRECOGNIZED ISCHEMIA OR INFARCTION

Both unrecognized ischemia and infarction may be present with symptoms that are mistakenly attributed to other organs (e.g. gastrointestinal problems). At least 8 percent to 10 percent of acute myocardial infarctions are painless (although not necessarily silent). Symptoms of ischemia or infarction may be typical or atypical.

The difference between ischemic and infarction pain is essentially a matter of degree. Ischemia is characteristically expressed by anterior chest discomfort (toward the center of the chest), like a tightness, constriction, indigestion, that lasts for a few minutes. An emotional upset or physical exertion usually provokes it. Resting or applying a nitroglycerin tablet under the tongue usually relieves it.

The pain of an acute myocardial infarction is typically described as a severe, knifelike pain, severe indigestion, a crushing sensation or pain or a choking discomfort. The pain may spread to both sides of the anterior thorax, the shoulder and arms, usually the left, with a tingling sensation that reaches the elbow, wrist and hand. Or it may affect the neck and jaw, the back, in between the shoulder blades. There is commonly associated nausea, vomiting, shortness of breath, profuse cold perspiration, dizziness, and weakness.

Other symptoms that are not as common may include abdominal pain that resembles acute gallbladder attack, peptic ulcer disease or pancreatitis, fainting, stroke, acute confusion and disorientation (particularly in the elderly), diarrhea, or the urge to defecate. I have seen patients with acute myocardial infarctions presenting *only* with pain in the right shoulder and arm, or *only* with pain in the jaw or the left ear lobe, or *only* with left elbow pain, or *only* with pain in the mid-abdominal region.

WHY SOME COMPLETE CORONARY OBSTRUCTIONS DO NOT CAUSE HEART ATTACKS

The process that leads to progressive blockage of a coronary artery usually takes months to years. This allows dormant vessels to dilate and serve a very useful function: They increase the blood supply to a neighboring affected, blood-deficient myocardial area.

The fact that collateral circulation develops is, in itself, an indication that a severe coronary artery obstruction exists, and it's usually blocking over 75 percent of the arterial lumen. These accessory vessels are extraordinarily important, because when the artery builds up a plaque that will eventually close off the vessel completely, the heart muscle territory in jeopardy will be protected by the collateral circulation system which supplies the necessary blood for the heart muscle's survival. So, curiously enough, and despite the total coronary artery obstruction, the myocardial infarction does not occur.

WHY QUICK ACTION IS NEEDED WHEN SYMPTOMS APPEAR

Approximately 1.1 million persons in the United States experience acute myocardial infarction annually. About 250,000 are instantly fatal. Of those who die, one-half do so within one hour of the onset of symptoms, before reaching the hospital. It is essential to seek emergent medical treatment as soon as possible when symptoms occur. Most of these fatal outcomes are due to ventricular fibrillation, a chaotic cardiac rhythm that can be converted to a normal one with an electrical discharge.

Well-equipped ambulances and helicopters staffed by trained personnel allow the initiation of treatment while a patient is being transported to the hospital. The effectiveness of this pre-hospital treatment depends on the competency of the paramedics, the radio-telemetry communication systems that allow transmission of electrocardiographic signals to the hospital, and the availability of specialized consultants who guide the initial and crucial therapeutic efforts.

Irreversible damage to the cardiac muscle occurs when the coronary artery has been completely occluded for about twenty minutes. Maximal damage occurs when the occlusion is sustained for four to six hours, but there is substantially greater salvage if restoration occurs in one to two hours. In selective cases, techniques to salvage myocardial tissue are implemented up to twelve hours after the beginning of persistent symptoms.

The use of thrombolytic drugs has improved the outcome of many heart attacks by dissolving the coronary clot (thrombus). However, not all acute myocardial infarctions qualify for this mode of therapy. Sometimes, the use of these agents may worsen the outcome. Your doctor knows which cases should (or should not) be managed with clot-dissolving drugs.

Right after his/her arrival at the hospital, the patient is treated with oxygen, morphine for pain relief, aspirin, intravenous nitroglycerin, beta-blockers, anti-arrhythmic drugs, etc., all of them, of course, applied according to each individual situation. Immediate consideration is given to the use of clot-dissolving drugs. Patients are carefully selected for this kind of treatment. Not every patient with an acute myocardial infarction should receive these medications. They may cause bleeding complication and other side-effects.

The good news is that we can do a lot about preventing and treating atherosclerosis. All we need to do is to acknowledge the seriousness of the issue, learn how to help ourselves, pay more attention to health-oriented literature, and pay less attention to the ads for unhealthy products.

It is essential to correct cardiovascular risk factors as much as possible, and make radical lifestyle changes. This is an absolute necessity for many people, and one that has been postponed for too long.

Appendix B
Cardiovascular Risk Factors

Sexuality and heart disease are complex issues. This complexity, though, does not prevent us from reaching a simple conclusion: Cardiovascular risk factors enhance the risk of cardiovascular disease, and cardiovascular disease increases the probability of sexual dysfunction. So, if you care about the latter, I urge you to pay careful attention to the former.

The American Heart Association recommends that assessment of cardiovascular risk begin at age 20 years, to be repeated at regular intervals.

It has been proposed that all apparently healthy men 45-75 years of age and women 55-75 years of age with no known history of coronary heart disease and who are considered not to be at very low risk undergo screening for atherosclerosis. Non-invasive screening tests for atherosclerosis are under investigation, and rapidly advancing, and include Magnetic Resonance Imaging (MRI) and Computerized Tomography (CT) for assessment of atherosclerotic plaques and detection of plaque inflammation. In addition, new serum biomarkers of inflammation in the arterial wall are being actively researched. At the present time, various modalities of stress tests, and scans for detection of calcium deposits in arteries are commonly employed.

Although some risk factors are unavoidable (age, gender, genes, and/or race), most heart attacks and strokes result from ignorance and lousy lifestyles. We are responsible for the excessive carbohydrates and fats we throw into our digestive system, eating toxic stuff at fast food chains, and taking our children with us-exposing them (unintentionally, of course) to the development of fatty streaks inside their tender arteries.

You are going to get older, because there's nothing you can do about the implacable stubbornness of the calendar. A healthy lifestyle, however, will make you feel good and keep you active for many years. If your genetic code flashes a red light of hypertension and high cholesterol levels, you can reduce or normalize them by appropriate medical management.

Our ability for self-destruction qualifies us for a medal. About 945,000 people die annually in the United States due to cardiovascular disease (heart attacks, strokes and hardening of the arteries), a number equivalent to the next eight leading causes of death combined, including cancer, chronic lung disease, AIDS, other infections, accidents, diabetes, suicides, and homicides. That number is quite close to the military casualties of all the United States wars since the Revolution.

Consider the possibility that you may have several risk factors threatening your heart right now. Review your nutrition, the time you spend daily with physical activities and regular exercise, and the degree of stress, depression, hostility, and/or anger you have to deal with every day. Ask yourself when was the last time you checked your cholesterol, blood pressure, and blood sugar. And finally, if your shirt smells of tobacco, you're definitely running behind schedule in the healthy heart game.

Age

The risk of heart disease increases with age. Of the 1.5 million myocardial infarctions that occur annually in the United States, only 75,000 affect people under 40.

Race

Coronary artery disease is the leading cause of death in African Americans. Whereas cardiovascular death rates have declined in the general American population over the past decade, death rates for African Americans have remained constant. African American women are at particular risk, with coronary heart disease rates 35 percent higher and stroke rates about 70 percent higher than rates for white women. This means that African Americans die younger, more suddenly, and more often than the general population.

African Americans are less likely than Whites to undergo cardiac catheterization, balloon dilatation of coronary arteries, and coronary bypass surgery.

Racial genetic influences have been advocated to explain the prevalence of cardio-vascular disease in the black population. What seems to be clear and more important than genetic differences between blacks and whites, is the constellation of social-economic problems that place African Americans at a disadvantage: low socio-economic status, education, occupation, social prejudice, inadequate medical care and health insurance-many being uninsured, others underinsured, all significantly contribute to poor control of obesity, high levels of cholesterol and triglycerides, hypertension, diabetes, etc. All of these conditions require adequate long-term care, follow-up, and adequate monitoring.

Family Background

If a parent or a sibling dies of a heart attack or hypertension complications before age 60, the risks of heart disease are higher for you.

Gender

Men are more likely than women to have coronary attacks before age 55. With advancing age, this difference becomes less significant and disappears by age 75, when the incidence of myocardial infarctions is similar in both sexes.

Lack of or Insufficient Information

People who lack sufficient information on basic health care issues, such as nutrition, physical activity, smoking, hypertension, and cholesterol, carry a higher risk for development of cardiovascular disease. Unfavorable socio-economic conditions and level of education play significant roles.

Mental/Emotional Road Blocks to Heart Health

Psychological-emotional dysfunctions can be important contributors to cardiovascular disease (coronary heart disease, hypertension, high cholesterol levels, or cardiac arrhythmias).

- Inability to set healthful priorities
- Denial about risk factors or disease
- Inconsistency in applying healthful routines
- Laziness
- Mental disorders (anxiety, depression, and others)
- Mental disorganization
- Poor self-discipline/will power

Abnormal Blood Lipids Levels

A low cholesterol-low triglyceride diet is essential to control lipids blood levels. Diet alone, though, is not always enough to get blood levels of total cholesterol, good cholesterol-HDL-, bad cholesterol-LDL-, and triglycerides below certain levels. The correction of *all* of these lipids fractions is very important. The currently recommended levels for cholesterol and LDL are about 20 mg/dl higher than those mentioned below. Many authorities feel that a more aggressive approach to the treatment of serum lipids should be recommended. For prevention, avoidance of progression, or even regression of coronary artery disease, they advise the following target numbers:

Total Cholesterol	Under 140 mg/dl
LDL (bad cholesterol)	Under 70 mg/dl
HDL (good cholesterol)	Over 50 mg/dl for men and over 55 mg/dl for women
Triglycerides	Under 130 mg %/dl

There are a number of medications to correct blood lipids abnormalities. The statin drugs (simvastatin, atorvastatin, lovastatin, etc.) are among the most important and effective.

Diabetes

This disease is a great promoter of cardiovascular disease and commonly leads to sexual dysfunction in both women and men. ED occurs because of penile arteries blockages due to atherosclerosis or diabetic neuropathy.

It is important to keep both the fasting blood glucose and postprandial (after meals) levels under control and an A1C glycohemoglobin level of 6 percent or less. A person who has diabetes should not have more than one drink a day (12 ounce can of beer or one 5-ounce glass of wine, or 1 ounce of 80-proof hard liquor.)

Reducing, or even better, normalizing body weight is extraordinarily important for the diabetic patient. Just too frequently, patients neglect this essential aspect of their treatment. Accompanying risk factors, such as hypertension, smoking, obesity, hyperlipidemia, must also be aggressively treated.

Unless there's a contraindication, ace-inhibitors (lisinopril, captopril, etc) or angiotensin blocking agents (losartan, etc) should be used. These drugs help to prevent or reduce the severity of vascular complications of diabetes, including renal failure.

The Metabolic Syndrome

The metabolic syndrome is diagnosed when 3 or more of the following 5 components are present:

- A waist circumference greater than 102 cm for men and more than 88 cm for women
- A fasting triglyceride level higher than 150 mg per dl
- A high-density lipoprotein (HDL) cholesterol level less than 40 mg per dl for men and less than 50 mg/dl for women
- Blood pressure higher than 135/80
- Fasting serum glucose concentration greater than 110 mg per dl

Data obtained from a 2000 census in the United States, estimated that 47 million people have the metabolic syndrome. If you estimate you have this syndrome, make an appointment with your healthcare practitioner and make plans to correct it.

Hypertension (Systolic and Diastolic)

Millions of individuals suffer from this condition without having the slightest idea about their existence and significance. Neglected hypertension kills. Before that happens, high blood pressure may cause chronic suffering and disability due to renal failure, congestive heart failure, heart attacks, strokes, and sexual dysfunction (SD).

Blood pressure (BP) above 115/70 increases the risk of cardiovascular complications. The risk is linear and doubles for each 20 mmg Hg systolic and 10 mm Hg diastolic BP elevations. These observations have lead to a new definition of pre-hypertension (systolic BP of 120-139 mm Hg or diastolic BP 80-89 mm Hg). Treatment of pre-hypertension has recently been shown to prevent the development of frank hypertension. The Journal of Clinical Hypertension reports that "Recent findings from large epidemiological studies indicate that the risks of cardiovascular disease may begin to increase at blood pressure levels well below 140/90, the current threshold for the definition and diagnosis of hypertension" (Thomas D. Giles, M.D., Aug 2006).

Management of high blood pressure requires the following:

- ♥ Achievement of normal weight
- ♥ Addressing alcohol use, sedentary lifestyle and obesity, as they contribute to resistant cases.
- ♥ Assessment of target organ damage (heart, brain, kidneys)
- ♥ Awareness of patient's sexual function prior to administration of any new antihypertensive drug
- ♥ Daily blood-pressure monitoring at home, with a record kept for future reference and therapeutic adjustments
- ♥ Good compliance taking medications as instructed; failure to do so, (poor compliance) is a frequent cause of complications and should be avoided
- ♥ Identification and correction of other cardiovascular risk factors. Hypertension usually has company (diabetes, obesity, dyslipidemia)
- ♥ Lifelong commitment to follow-up and treatment is needed
- ♥ Monitoring possible side effects of medications

- ❤ Reduction of salt intake
- ❤ Screening for possible curable causes, such as blockage of renal artery, among others, when   necessary
- ❤ Selection of antihypertensive drug or drugs based on patient's age, state of nutrition, weight, and concomitant illnesses
- ❤ Stress control and suppression of chronic upsetting situations, if possible.

Left Ventricular Hypertrophy

This condition represents the increased thickness of the left ventricular walls that may result from hypertension and other causes. It is considered another important cardiovascular risk factor since it is associated with higher incidence of malignant cardiac rhythm disturbances and sudden death.

Smoking

Smoking is the single most important factor for both women and men. Smoking is a deadly poison. It is *really* bad. And it is difficult for many smokers to understand that something that gives them so much pleasure can be so destructive. What makes this habit particularly tragic is that it is totally preventable. Every year, 400,000 people die in the United States from smoking. Secondhand smoking causes another 57,000 deaths annually, of which 37,000 are due to cardiovascular disease. In Europe, smoking is responsible for 1.2 million burials every year.

Tobacco contains over 2,000 gases and chemicals, some of which damage the cardiovascular system and lead to cancer. Nicotine, carbon monoxide, and polycyclic aromatic hydrocarbons are just a few of them. There is no evidence that filters or other cigarette modifications reduce risks. Low tar, low nicotine cigarettes do not solve the problem either.

Cigar and pipe smokers live with the delusion that this kind of smoking is not harmful. The reason for this, they say, is that they do not inhale. Their lungs, however, inhale the smoke that hangs around them anyway. Their blood levels of nicotine or a nicotine-derivative-the urine cotinin level-are at times as high as that of cigarette smokers. Cigars contain more tobacco than cigarettes. A cigarette is smoked in about six minutes. A cigar takes much longer, and the oral and respiratory exposure to its toxins is significant.

Smoking and its by-products enter the body by two different paths: through inhalation, and through the mouth. The former (inhalation) leads to lung and larynx cancer, and the latter (via the mouth) is a precursor of cancer of the tongue, lips, throat, esophagus, and stomach. There is also a strong correlation between smoking and pancreatic cancer. Some of the side affects of smoking:

- Constriction of coronary and cerebral arteries
- Damage to the inner layer of arteries (endothelium)
- Impotence and erectile failure
- Increase in blood clotting; promotes blood fibrinogen and platelet adhesiveness
- Increases the damaging influence of other cardiovascular risk factors
- Increases the number of heart attacks and strokes
- Destroys lungs(chronic bronchitis and emphysema)
- Causes multiple cancers
- Promotes nicotine addiction
- Obstructs multiple arteries, including those that supply blood to the genitals and lower extremities
- Reduces blood levels of "good" HDL (high-density lipoprotein) cholesterol, which is cardio-protective; increases blood levels of "bad" LDL (low-density lipoprotein) cholesterol, which is coronary unfriendly
- Promotes thromboangiitis, a very painful and disabling disorder of the circulation of the legs that affects male smokers almost exclusively
- Worsens symptoms of cold hands and feet in those who suffer a vascular disorder called Raynaud's disease

Quitting smoking is essential. Nicotine patches and nicotine gums help and can be used in combination with Wellbutrin, a prescription medication your doctor can prescribe. The one-year success rate of these agents, when used combined, is at best 35%.

Sedentary Lifestyle

Watching television many hours a day, or sitting in front of a computer for endless hours, have become occupational hazards. Currently, 75 percent of the United States' adult population does not exercise regularly. Women and the elderly tend to be less active. The U.S. Centers for Disease Control and Prevention estimated that 250,000 deaths occur each year in the USA due to lack of exercise. Yet exercise-done properly and regularly-reduces the risk of cardiovascular events in both sexes by 50 percent, and lowers the risk of adult-onset diabetes and cancers of the breast, ovaries, prostate, and colon.

It's important not to confuse leanness with fitness. Leanness means to be not fat or fleshy. Fitness means a healthy physical response to exercise. A recent study, which involved nearly 21,000 men followed during an eight-year period, reported a much higher incidence of cardiovascular-related death in *lean*, unfit men than in men who were obese but fit.

The health benefits of exercise extend to more than the cardiovascular areas. Regular exercise helps control anxiety and depression, raises levels of good cholesterol (HDL), keeps the muscles toned and in shape, preserves bone mass, enhances physical coordination, and gives you a sense of well-being. However, be careful about vigorous physical activity and avoid it, unless you are physically prepared *and* your doctor approves it. The risk of cardiac arrest increases fivefold during strenuous efforts. The risk of dying from a sedentary lifestyle, however, is twice as high.

Abdominal Obesity

Abdominal obesity is considered a major cardiovascular risk factor for coronary and cardiovascular mortality in men and women. In general, the fatter the belly, the greater the risk. In adults with severe abdominal obesity, the risk of developing coronary artery disease increases almost nine-fold. Strokes are also a part of the cardiovascular risk package. Although there are health risks associated with obesity in general, these are more closely correlated with distribution of body fat, rather than total amount.

One-third of the United States population is obese, and the prevalence of obesity is increasing. The way an abdomen becomes obese varies from person to person. It may be a result of anxiety, depression, low socioeconomic conditions, social-occupational situations, genetic influences (familial obesity), drugs (oral contraceptives, steroids, and some antihypertensive agents, such as beta-blockers and clonidine), an under-active thyroid (hypothyroidism), or even an injury.

Attempts to correct abdominal obesity require making a clear decision to be firm and consistent following a new food and exercise plan. Once you get used to consuming the proper foods, limiting your caloric intake, and doing regular, consistent exercise, you will noticeably see the results, and eliminate this risk.

Low Birth Weight

Studies done in India, the United States, and the United Kingdoms have shown that low birth weight is associated with an increased risk of coronary artery disease, heart attacks, hypertension, strokes, and other conditions (diabetes, renal failure, and thyroid disorders) in adult life. The incidence of coronary artery disease among men and women over 45 years of age whose birth weight was less than 5.5 pounds was 11 percent, as opposed to a 3 percent incidence among those whose birth weight was greater than seven pounds. The highest rate of coronary artery disease (20 percent) was observed among people whose birth weight was less than 5.5 pounds and whose mothers weighed less than 100 pounds.

Socioeconomic conditions, poverty, malnutrition, and poor prenatal care are some of the reasons for low birth weights. Additionally, there are other causes for premature births (where birth weight is necessarily low) and of course, these happen at any socioeconomic level.

Chronic Infections and Inflammations

A number of studies carried out in the United States and other countries for the past several years offer highly suggestive evidence about the possible role of chronic infections in the production of atherosclerotic lesions, recurrent, unstable angina, and myocardial infarctions. *Chlamydia pneumoniae,* a germ often found in patients suffering from chronic bronchitis, is a prime suspect. Currently, it is believed that this organism is responsible for about 10 percent of the community-acquired pneumonias and 5 percent of bronchitis and sinusitis episodes. It is also clear that *C. pneumoniae* has an affinity for atherosclerotic plaques. There are other germs that are thought to be responsible for the development of obstructive plaques inside the arterial system.

C-Reactive Protein is a marker of inflammation. Lately, CRP has been a source of growing interest and concern. Although it may show elevated blood levels during infections due to C. Pneumoniae and other infectious organisms, it is also elevated during inflammatory processes where there is no infection, such as rheumatoid arthritis, lupus and ulcerative colitis. Levels of CRP can also be elevated when there is no discernable cause. The presence of abnormally high levels of CRP, and its inflammatory action, renders atherosclerotic plaques more vulnerable to rupture and the consequent development of an acute myocardial infarction.

Psychosocial Factors

Chronic stress resulting from a number of socio-economic problems, cultural-religious conflicting couples' relationships, reduced income, unemployment, may contribute in varying degrees to the development and perpetuation of cardiovascular disorders, such as coronary heart disease, hypertension, and strokes. See Depression for more information.

Alcohol

Alcohol is the most widely used drug in the United States. In a way, it is also the most predictable. We know that the effects of alcohol on the heart (and other areas as well) are dose-dependent.

There is no question that the chronic use of alcohol may cause disease of the heart muscle (alcoholic cardiomyopathy). The cardiac chambers become dilated and flabby. The contractile power of the heart is badly affected. The pump loses strength. This results in congestive heart failure, accumulation of fluid in various regions of the body, clots inside the heart which can travel to the brain or other places (clots form because the blood flow inside the heart is sluggish in a very enlarged heart), and arrhythmias of all types, some of them life-threatening. Acute alcohol consumption is also a well known cause of cardiac arrhythmias called "the holiday syndrome."

There is also a link between alcohol abuse and hypertension. High stroke rates, particularly cerebral hemorrhages, are seen in alcoholics. In fact, the risk of stroke in alcoholics increases threefold.

In chronic hypertensive patients, it is very important to limit or eliminate alcohol consumption, because it may interfere with the effectiveness of drug therapy. Once alcohol is removed from the picture, the blood pressure usually takes just a few days to improve or normalize.

The purely medical consequences of alcohol include liver cirrhosis, jaundice, confusion, infections, gastrointestinal bleeding, bone-marrow depression, anemia, impotence, and breast enlargement (gynecomastia) and feminine-like hip development in men. Alcohol also causes sodium retention due to stimulation of cortisone secretion by the adrenal gland. This results in higher blood pressure and potassium loss, both of which can trigger cardiac arrhythmias. It also acts as a diuretic and leads to dehydration due to fluid loss, thus increasing blood clotting tendencies and myocardial infarctions.

Alcohol use during pregnancy may seriously damage the fetus with various physical deformities and mental retardation (called fetal alcohol syndrome and fetal alcohol effects), and may even cause fetal death.

Alcohol does not give you a good, flexible, healthy margin to work with. If you drink very little, it's good for you. Alcohol helps raise good HDL cholesterol levels, and thus may offer some protection against atherosclerosis. One drink a day is ideal. Two drinks a day is the maximum to be consumed, as long as each drink contains no more than one ounce of alcohol. Two drinks a day equals two ounces of hard liquor (rum, gin, scotch, whiskey or vodka) or two, five-ounces glasses of wine, or two twelve-ounce cans of beer. If you drink more than you should, be prepared for trouble.

These small amounts are associated with a 30 to 50 percent reduction in the risk of developing coronary artery disease. The risk for stroke is reduced by 50 percent. These benefits apply to all alcoholic beverages, not just red wine.

- It raises the levels of HDL, the protective cholesterol
- It reduces the tendency for blood clotting. This "anticoagulant" effect is more effective when alcohol is consumed with meals, because the tendency to clot formation in the circulation is increased after eating
- Some alcohol products, such as red and white wine, contain flavonoid antioxidants that reduce the oxidation of LDL, the coronary *unfriendly* cholesterol

Despite the potential benefits of alcohol in small amounts on the cardiovascular system, this substance is not recommended to reduce the risk of heart attacks or strokes. For those who can control the amount of alcohol they drink, one or two drinks a day in the recommended doses may be acceptable.

Individuals with alcohol addiction should seek immediate specialized counseling, and avoid drinking even one drop of alcohol for the rest of their lives.

Blood Abnormalities

Any one of a number of abnormal blood conditions can increase an individual's risk for coronary artery disease and heart attack. Included among these are:

- Increased numbers of red blood cells
- Increased white blood cells
- Increased platelets
- Dysfunctional platelets
- Increased levels of fibrinogen
- Increased levels of Lipoprotein(a)
- Increased homocysteine levels

Other Conditions

Some medical conditions and drug therapies may put an individual at increased risk for heart disease. These include:

- AIDS
- Birth-control pill usage by smokers or those who have hypertension
- Long-term estrogen therapy
- Hypothyroidism (under-active thyroid)
- Long-standing estrogen deficiency in women
- Prolonged treatment with cortisone-derivatives and androgenic steroids
- Some chronic kidney diseases
- Systemic lupus
- Transplanted heart
- Vascular disease in extra-cardiac vascular territories-for example, carotid artery disease or peripheral-vascular disease (arteriosclerosis of lower extremity arteries)

Cocaine

In 1884, cocaine was first introduced into medical practice as a local anesthetic. For quite a while, cocaine was thought to be a safe and nonaddicting agent. The increase in the recreational use of this substance, however, suggested otherwise. In fact, people died from using it. More than six million Americans now use cocaine regularly.

The pharmaceutical extract has a purity of 89 percent. "Street" cocaine, on the other hand, is usually mixed with adulterants (lactose, quinine, etc.), which results in a purity of anywhere from 25 percent to 90 percent. Pure cocaine is insoluble in water and can be extracted from "street" cocaine by using an alkaline solution and an organic solvent. When this solvent mixture evaporates, a purified alkaloid rock results. This is called "crack" cocaine, because of the characteristic sound it produces when heated.

Cocaine can be injected intravenously or inhaled into the lungs-which produces a "quick high" that last from 20 to 30 minutes. Intranasal use ("snorting") results in a delayed onset of action, and the cocaine is absorbed more slowly. The accompanying euphoria lasts from 60 to 90 minutes.

Acute myocardial infarction is the most frequent cardiac complication of cocaine use. It is due to severe constriction of a coronary artery and/or to the cocaine-induced increased tendency to form blood clots. Taking into consideration the large numbers of cocaine users, these complications are probably infrequent. I once treated a twenty-three-year-old athletic boy who had sustained a very extensive acute myocardial infarction due to cocaine. He survived, although his heart muscle was badly damaged. Several months later, as he was trying to make a new life for himself, his family found him dead in bed.

The dose of consumed cocaine does not appear to be the related to heart attacks. Both small doses of street cocaine (as little as 25 to 50 mg) have caused heart attacks, as have massive doses (1.5 grams). Other deadly complications of cocaine consumption are: sudden death preceded by delirium, high fever, anxiety, panic, seizures, and violence. Cerebral and aortic aneurysms have ruptured following acute cocaine-induced

Alcoholism, Cocaine, HIV, and Heart Disease: An Explosive Cocktail

David was a 25-year-old homosexual receiving multiple medications for AIDS. He had been an alcoholic since childhood, was a heavy smoker and a cocaine addict, and barely survived a cocaine-induced, acute, extensive myocardial infarction. His two sisters and six brothers were alcoholic. Since it is unusual to see all siblings suffering from alcoholism, I inquired about the reasons. David told me his parents died young, and his grandmother raised the nine children, plus six other orphans. According to David, "She went crazy every night with all the kids' screaming and crying. So she silenced all of us with bottles of beer instead of milk."

Soon after his heart attack, David was found dead in bed.

Being a physician is not enough to solve problems like this. You need to be a magician.

hypertension. Pulmonary edema (excessive fluid in the lungs), although not cardiac-related, has also been observed.

CONCLUSION

Do you have any of these risk factors If you live in the United States or any Western country, and you *don't* have any cardiovascular risk factors, it's a miracle.

Try to beat coronary disease before it begins-or progresses further. Make a list of your risks, by first identifying those you know you have, and then making a secondary list of those you suspect you have. Then, speak to your physician to find out those you didn't know you have.

As far as the preservation of your sexual function is concerned, I urge you to review these risk factors until you are convinced that you've rid yourself of as many of them as you can. Even a single risk factor may disrupt your life.

Appendix C

Practical Tips on Commonly Used Cardiac Drugs

ACE INHIBITORS (ANGIOTENSIN-CONVERTING-ENZYME INHIBITORS)

Examples: benazepril, captopril, enalapril, lisinopril, ramipril

These drugs are very effective in the treatment of hypertension. They also slow the progression of vascular disease—for example, damage to the kidneys and retinas in diabetic patients. Additionally, they have proved extremely valuable in the management of chronic heart failure and in the treatment of acute myocardial infarction. (Treatment starts within the first twenty-four to thirty-six hours of the acute heart attack and continues for one year or longer if necessary.) Studies have documented a significant reduction in acute myocardial infarction complications in both patients who have had an acute, uncomplicated myocardial infarction, and in those who have damaged the myocardium and are left with a weakened cardiac muscle.

It is important to monitor renal function when ACE inhibitors are used to ensure that they do not cause excessive blood pressure reduction (hypotension).

A dry cough occurs in five to ten percent of patients on ACE inhibitors (more frequently seen in women), and usually requires the discontinuation of the drug.

ALDACTONE (SPIRONOLACTONE)

Aldosterone is a hormone synthesized by the adrenal gland that is now recognized as responsible for a number of adverse effects on the cardiovascular system. It

253

impairs the production of nitric oxide by the endothelium, damages the inner layer of the arteries, and promotes blood clotting by inhibiting the degradation of fibrin (a substance that contributes to clot formation). Additionally, data accumulated for the past ten years shows that aldosterone produces myocardial fibrosis-scarring of the heart muscle-which makes it weak).

Aldosterone antagonism-that is, "neutralizing" the effects of aldosterone-is currently the cornerstone of therapy for patients with congestive heart failure, together with other agents such as ace inhibitors, angiotensin receptor blockers, and beta-blockers. The drug that neutralizes aldosterone is called spironolactone (Aldactone). It occasionally causes some enlargement and tenderness of the breasts. Understandably, the possibility of this side effect creates more concern for males. The effect disappears, however, when the medication is discontinued.

ANGIOTENSIN II RECEPTOR BLOCKERS

Examples: losartan, valsartan

Indications for these drugs are quite similar to those for the ACE inhibitors. ARBs, however, do not produce a dry cough.

ASPIRIN

In 2002, the American Heart Association issued an update on Aspirin therapy for primary prevention of cardiovascular disease and stroke. A low daily dose of 75-160 mg appears to be just as effective as higher doses.

The American Diabetes Association now recommends aspirin therapy for prevention of heart attacks or strokes in diabetic patients who have an additional risk factor, such as high blood pressure or smoking.

Aspirin should not be taken by patients with aspirin intolerance or aspirin allergy, or by those at increased risk for gastrointestinal or intra-cerebral bleeding.

The effects of Aspirin vary among individuals and this might explain, in part, why patients receiving Aspirin therapy still carry a relatively high risk of recurrent vascular events.

254

Aspirin resistance is an elusive diagnosis, difficult to establish in a formal way, but it is generally described as the failure of Aspirin to prevent blood clotting inside the arteries. It has been suspected to have an incidence of 5 percent to 45 percent of the general population.

BETA-BLOCKERS

Examples: acebutolol, atenolol, betaxolol, carvedilol, metoprolol, nadolol, pindolol, propranolol, sotalol, timolol

These drugs interfere with the effects of adrenaline-like hormones that normally increase heart rate and blood pressure. They are very effective in the management of angina. They also decrease the workload of the heart and slow the heart rate. Additionally, beta-blockers are useful in treating hypertension, some cases of heart failure, and cardiac rhythm disturbances (arrhythmias). Some are also prescribed for a condition called familial tremor, as well as for hyperthyroidism (overactive thyroid) and for the management of migraines and glaucoma.

Adverse side effects of beta-blockers include excessive bradycardia (slow heart rate), bronchospasm and aggravation of wheezing, depression, vivid dreams, constipation, and erectile failure. In patients who have diabetes and are on insulin, the symptoms of hypoglycemia may be masked by beta-blockers.

CALCIUM CHANNEL BLOCKERS OR CALCIUM ANTAGONISTS

Examples: amlodipine, diltiazem, felodipine, nifedipine, verapamil

These drugs are commonly used for the treatment of angina and hypertension. They act by dilating the arteries, which leads to increased blood flow and lowering of blood pressure. Side effects include headaches, flushing, leg edema, constipation, and excessive drop in blood pressure. There are rare reports of sexual dysfunction attributed to these medications.

NITROGLYCERIN AND NITRATE DERIVATIVES

The first-line therapy for patients with angina/angina pectoris is self-administration of sublingual nitroglycerin tablets (0.3 to 0.6 mg), or an equivalent oral spray (with each puff delivering approximately 0.4 mg). Because nitroglycerin tablets lose their potency over time, it is preferable to keep only a two- to three-month supply on hand. It is also advisable to carry just a few with you and keep the remainder in small brown bottles in the refrigerator. The brown containers protect the tablets from sunlight, which causes the tablets to lose potency at a much faster pace.

The oral nitroglycerin spray provides over 200 aerosol doses of 0.4 mg, has a shelf life of two years or more, and does not require refrigeration.

For chronic and mild angina that occurs less than once a week, sublingual nitroglycerin may be enough to keep symptoms in check. However, beta-blockers, calcium channel blockers, and long-acting nitrates are usually indicated when angina occurs more often-particularly when hypertension is present. These medications not only help relieve angina, but they lower blood pressure as well.

Nitroglycerin can also be administered in other formulations, including a slow-acting, dissolving oral capsule, and through the skin. This latter method is called "transdermal", and it's applied as an ointment or a patch. Intravenous nitroglycerin is frequently used in the hospital setting for severe, acute, unstable coronary insufficiency.

A common mistake made by patients who use sublingual nitroglycerin is the failure to take it *preventively*—that is, before physical exertions and/or events that are known to precipitate chest pains, *including sexual activity*. Discuss taking nitroglycerin preventively with your physician.

One disadvantage of long-term nitrate therapy (using nitroglycerin and nitrate-derivatives) is the development of tolerance to the medication. A decreased response to nitroglycerin is often seen when a nitrate compound is regularly given without an eight- to twelve-hour nitrate-free interval. These medication-free periods may be prescribed during the day or during the night. Your physician will advise you on the preferred hours to abstain from your long-acting nitroglycerin or nitrate-derivative. In some instances, it is important that you be protected with a beta-blocker or a calcium channel blocker during the nitroglycerin-free or nitrate-derivative-free hours.

256

Nitroglycerin patches should be used for twelve hours and removed for twelve hours.

Sublingual nitroglycerin tablets can be taken up to three times, five minutes apart, for chest pain due to angina, for those who tolerate the medication well without significant dizziness or headaches. Get your doctor's advice on this too. While there are patients who have good tolerance to nitroglycerin, others faint and collapse after taking just one tablet. Other common side effects include flushing and headaches.

Concomitant use of aspirin may prevent or minimize headaches and also prevent coronary events.

10 percent of patients prescribed nitroglycerin or nitrate-derivatives will not be able to take these medications because of severe headaches.

The beneficial action of nitroglycerin and nitrate-derivatives in relieving angina results from two effects on the circulation:

Coronary artery dilation and increased blood flow to a myocardium (heart muscle) that needs better blood supply, and,

A venous-dilating effect on the large body veins that allows for some pooling of blood and a reduction of venous return to the heart chambers. This reduces the work of the heart which results in improvement or avoidance of an angina attack.

WATER

There is some evidence suggesting that water can be cardio-protective and reduce the risk of heart attacks. In one study, thousands of men and women who drank five or more glasses of water a day had a significantly lower risk of fatal heart attack and stroke.

Why would water have these beneficial effects? Perhaps because of its diluting effect on the blood, which makes the blood less viscous and therefore less prone to clot formation. Other beneficial effects may include the diluting effects of proper hydration on the adhesiveness of platelets; better elimination through the kidneys of substances circulating in the blood that are pro-clotting; or the content of calcium and magnesium in hard waters. Calcium and magnesium have been associated with lower death rates from coronary artery disease and decreased risk of fatal arrhythmias following a heart attack.

Commonly Recommended Nitrate Regimens for
Chronic Stable Angina*

*For practical purposes, blanks are intentional

Preparation	Dosage	Time to Peak	Duration of Action
Nitroglycerin Sublingual tablet or spray	.3-.4 mg	2 minutes	25 minutes
Oral Sustained-Released nitroglycerin	2.5-6.5 mg capsules every 12 hours	35 minutes	4 hours
Isosorbide Mononitrate Sublingual		15 minutes	1 hour
Isosorbide Mononitrate Rapid release	20 mg in AM, 20 mg 7 hr later	12-14 hours	
Isosorbide Mononitrate Sustained release	120-140 mg a day		10-12 hours
Isosorbide Dinitrate Sublingual		15 minutes	1 hour
Isosorbide Dinitrate Rapid release	30 mg twice daily at 7 AM and 1 PM		6 hours
Isosorbide Dinitrate Oral sustained release		75 minutes	12 hours
Nitroglycerin patches applied to the skin	7.5-10 mg for 12 hours		10-12 hours

Resources

BOOKS ON CORONARY HEART DISEASE: NUTRITION, REVERSAL METHODS, AND PREVENTION

Chapunoff, Eduardo, M.D. *Morbid Obesity and the Struggle for Survival.* iUniverse. Lincoln, NE: 2007.

Gersh, Bernard J., M.D. *Mayo Clinic Heart Book, Revised Edition.* William Morrow. New York: 2002.

Gould, K. Lance, M.D. *Heal Your Heart: How You Can Prevent or Reverse Heart Disease.* Rutgers University Press. Piscataway, NJ: 1998.

Mogadam, Michael, M.D. *Every Heart Attack is Preventable.* Lifeline Press. Washington, D.C.: 2003.

Robbins, John. *The Food Revolution.* Conary Press. Berkeley, CA: 2001.

BOOKS ON PROBLEM-SOLVING METHODS FOR PERSONAL AND RELATIONSHIP CONFLICTS

Fay, Allen, M.D. *Making It as a Couple: Prescription for a Quality Relationship.* FMC Books. Essex, CT: 1999.

Fay, Allen, M.D., Lazarus, Arnold, Ph.D. *I Can If I Want To.* FMC Books. Essex, CT.: 2000.

Lazarus, Arnold, Ph.D., Lazarus, Clifford, Ph.D. *The 60-Second Shrink: Over 100 strategies for Staying Sane in a Crazy World.* Barnes & Noble Books. New York: 1999.

BOOKS ON SEXUALITY

Masters, William H., Johnson, Virginia E., and Kolodny, Robert C. *Human Sexuality.* HarperCollins. New York: 1997.

Reinisch, June M., Ph.D. *The Kinsey Institute: New Report on Sex.* St. Martin's Press. New York: 1994.

Stoppard, Miriam, M.D. *The Magic of Sex.* Dorling Kindersley. New York: 2001.

Yaffe, Maurice and Fenwick, Elizabeth. *Sexual Happiness for Women.* Henry Holt and Company. New York: 1992.

Comfort, Alex, M.D. *The Joy of Sex.* Pocket Books. New York: 2004.

AGENCIES
Aging
National Institutes on Aging

P. O. Box 8057

Gaithersburg, MD 20898-8057

1-800-222-2225

National Council on Aging

409 Third Street SW, Suite 200

Washington, DC 20024

1-800-424-9046

Alcohol
1-800-ALCOHOL

This hot line is available twenty-four hours a day, seven days a week. Offers counseling and assistance in finding local treatment centers.

Alcoholics Anonymous, Inc.

General Service Office

P. O. Box 459

Grand Central Station

New York, NY 10163

212-870-3400

Cardiovascular Health
American Heart Association
National Center

7272 Greenview Avenue

Dallas, Tx 75231-4596

800-242-8721

National Heart, Lung, and Blood Institute
Information Center

P. O. Box 30105

Bethesda, MD 20824-0105

301-251-1222

Sudden Arrhythmia Death Syndrome Foundation
P. O. Box 58767

Salt Lake City, UT 84158

Diabetes
American Diabetes Association, Inc.
1660 Duke Street

Alexandria, VA 22314

800-232-3472

National Diabetes Information Clearinghouse
One Information Way

Bethesda, MD 20892-3560

301-654-3327

Drugs
National Institute on Drug Abuse
1-800-662-4357

Narcotics Anonymous
www.na.org.

General Health Services and Information
National Library of Medicine
8600 Rockville Pike

Bethesda, MD 20894

1-800-272-4787

Mental Health Organizations
The National Mental Health Association
www.nmha.org
Mental Health Net–Self Help Source Book
mentalhelp.net/selfhelp

Nutrition
National Center for Nutrition and Dietetics (NCND)
216 West Jackson Boulevard, Suite 800

Chicago, IL 60606-6995

1-800-366-1655
National Cholesterol Education Program
NHLBI Information Center

P. O. Box 30105

Bethesda, MD 20824-0105

301-251-1222
Seafood Hotline
U.S. Food and Drug Administration

1-800-332-4010

Sexual Dysfunction
Female Impotence
www.healthfind.org/health/female+impotence

Impotence Institute of America

800-669-1603

www.impotenceworld.orq.

Sexuality
The Society for the Scientific Study of Sexuality

P. O .Box 416

Allentown, PA 18105-0416

Phone: 610-530-2483

Fax: 610-530-2485

Website: www.SexScience.org

Smoking
American Cancer Society

National Office

1599 Clifton Road NE

Atlanta, GA 30329

1-800-ACS-2345

American Lung Association

1740 Broadway, 14th Floor

New York, NY 10019-4374

1-800-586-4872

American Heart Association

National Center

7320 Greenville Avenue

Dallas, TX 75231

1-800-AHA-USA1

Stroke

National Institute of Neurological Disorders and Stroke

NINDS Information Service

Building 31, Room 8, A06

Bethesda, MD 20892

301-496-5751

National Stroke Association

300 East Hampden Avenue, Suite 200

Englewood, CO 80110-2622

1-800-787-6537

American Stroke Association

Phone: 1-888-478-7653

Fax: 214-706-5231

Glossary

abdominal angina: Abdominal discomfort caused by obstruction of an artery that supplies blood to the intestines.

ablation: Removal or elimination of a localized area of cardiac muscle responsible for causing severe tachycardia. There are several ablation techniques. A common one is "radiofrequency ablation". It is done by introducing wires (catheters) inside the cardiac chambers through the groin blood vessels.

alcoholic heart disease: Weakening of the heart muscle caused by chronic, excessive alcohol consumption (alcoholic cardiomyopathy) which may produce congestive heart failure, arrhythmias, or both.

amiodarone: Drug used to reverse or control significant cardiac arrhythmias.

angina: Chest pain or discomfort due to deficient blood supply to the heart muscle. Sometimes called angina pectoris.

aneurysm: Potentially life-threatening blood-filled bulge of a blood vessel, particularly an artery, which may occur in one of many arterial areas in the body. These include the brain (a brain-cerebral aneurysm); the thorax (a thoracic aortic aneurysm); the heart (a coronary artery aneurysm); the abdomen (an abdominal aortic aneurysm);, and the groin (an iliac artery aneurysm), among others.

angiogram (angiography): X-ray picture of arteries that have been injected with a radio-opaque substance that allows them to be seen and analyzed. If the coronary arteries are investigated, the test is called a coronary angiogram.

angioplasty: Treatment of an arterial atherosclerotic plaque that severely narrows the vessel by the use of a wire (catheter) that has a balloon at its tip. This is positioned at the level of the blockage and when it is dilated, it relieves the obstruction, and restores blood flow.

angiotensin II receptor antagonist: Drug used for hypertension and heart failure.

angiotensin-converting enzyme (ACE) inhibitor: A drug that lowers the blood pressure and is very helpful in the management of heart failure, cardiomyopathies, and hypertension.

antianginal drug: Any drug used to prevent or relieve anginal pain or discomfort.

anticoagulant: A blood thinner. Any drug that prevents blood clotting or delays it.

antihypertensive: Any drug or other therapy that lowers the blood pressure.

Antiplatelet medications: Reduce risk of blood clots, which might contribute to unstable angina, heart attack, or stroke.

aorta: The largest artery in the body, it originates in the left ventricle of the heart and carries blood to the rest of the body.

aortic valve: One of four heart valves, the aortic valve is located at the exit of the left ventricle of the heart where the aorta begins. It allows blood to be pumped out to aorta. *See also* aorta, left ventricle

arrhythmia (dysrrhythmia): Abnormal heart beat (slow, fast, or irregular).

arterial spasm: Constriction of an artery.

arteritis: Inflammation of the artery.

artery, arteries: Blood vessels that carry fresh, oxygenated blood throughout the body.

arteriosclerosis: Hardening of the arteries. The process is caused by an atheroma in the inner layer of the artery, plus reactions in other layers of the vessel. *See also* atheroma, atherosclerosis

ascending aorta: The first portion of the aorta, emerging from the heart's left ventricle.

atherectomy: A non-surgical procedure for treating diseased arteries with a rotating device that shaves away obstructing material inside the artery.

atheroma: Localized fatty material that forms a plaque inside the arteries. When the coronary artery is affected and the lumen of the vessel is narrowed significantly, a myocardial infarction may result. Heart attacks most often result from small, soft, moderately obstructive coronary plaques, which crack and allow the immediate formation of a clot that then blocks the artery completely.

atherogenic: Any material that contributes to the formation of atherosclerotic plaques.

atherosclerosis: A process of atheroma formation that primarily affects the inner layer of an artery. The reaction that involves the other layers of the artery causes hardening of the vessel's wall and that is called arteriosclerosis. *See also* arteriosclerosis

atrial fibrillation: A rhythm characterized by disorganized contractions of the atrial muscle and that has replaced the normal cardiac rhythm producing an irregular heart beat.

atrium: *See* left atrium, right atrium.

beta-blocker: A drug used for treatment of hypertension, angina, arrhythmias, cardiomyopathies, migraine headaches, and familial tremor.

blood pressure: Pressure or force exerted by the blood inside the arteries, resulting from the heart's pumping action.

bradycardia: Abnormally slow heartbeat

bruit: An abnormal sound heard when the stethoscope is applied over a narrowed, diseased artery. It is particularly useful in detecting carotid artery disease.

calcium-channel blocker (calcium blocker): A drug used for treatment of hypertension, angina, and arrhythmias.

cardiac: Pertaining to the heart.

cardiac arrest: The stopping of the heart beat.

cardiac catheterization: A procedure that involves the insertion of a fine tube (catheter) into an artery, usually in the groin area, and passing the tube into the heart. It is done under local anesthesia. It evaluates the status of the heart function and valves and it is usually used in conjunction with the coronary angiogram, which identifies obstructions of coronary arteries, their precise locations and severity. It is often an indispensable tool in the diagnosis and treatment of heart disease.

cardiac output: The amount of blood the heart pumps through the circulatory system in one minute.

cardiac transplantation: Replacement of a very defective heart with one of a donor.

cardiology: Study of the heart and its function in health and disease.

cardiomyopathy: A disease of the heart muscle that often results in deterioration of the heart's pumping ability.

cardiovascular system: It consists of the heart and all the blood vessels (arteries and veins) that circulate blood throughout the body.

cardioversion: A technique of applying an electrical shock to the chest in an attempt to convert an abnormal cardiac rhythm to a normal one.

carotid artery: A major artery (right and left) in the neck supplying blood to the brain.

cerebral embolism: A blood clot that is carried by the bloodstream to the brain, where it blocks an artery.

cerebral hemorrhage: Bleeding within the brain resulting from a ruptured blood vessel, aneurysm, or a head injury.

cerebral thrombosis: Formation of a blood clot inside an artery that supplies blood to the brain.

cerebrovascular accident: An impeded blood supply to some part of the brain, resulting in damage to the brain tissue. *See also* stroke

cholesterol: One of many fatty substances that circulate in the blood stream and contribute to atherosclerosis. *See also* high-density lipoprotein, lipoproteins, low-density lipoprotein, triglycerides, and very-low-density lipoprotein

claudication: A tireness or pain in the arms, thighs or legs caused by inadequate blood supply caused by diseased, narrowed, arteriosclerotic arteries.

coronary arteries: Vessels that supply blood to the heart. They reach all portions of the cardiac muscle giving the appearance of a crown-like structure. Coronary derives from the Latin corona, meaning crown.

collateral circulation: New blood vessels that grow following a significant chronic obstruction of a coronary artery; they carry blood to the heart muscle beyond the blocked arterial segment and act as a natural bypass mechanism.

conduction system: Special bundles that conduct electrical impulses throughout the muscle of the heart.

congestive heart failure: Weakened heart muscle resulting in fluid accumulation in the lungs and other organs.

coronary artery disease: Narrowing of coronary arteries by atherosclerotic plaques.

coronary bypass surgery: "Bridge" created by a segment of vein removed from the leg or arm that connects the aorta to a coronary artery below a severe coronary artery obstruction (venous bypass graft) or a thoracic artery called internal mammary artery (internal mammary bypass graft).

cyanosis: Blueness of skin caused by insufficient oxygen in the blood.

coronary heart disease: Symptoms (angina, for example) and/or events (a myocardial infarction, for example), that occur because of coronary artery disease. Also called ischemic heart disease. *See also* ischemia

deep-vein thrombosis (DVT): A blood clot formed in a deep vein, usually in one of the lower extremities veins.

diastole: Each cardiac expansion (dilation) and relaxation. *See also* systole.

diastolic blood pressure: The lowest blood pressure measured in the arteries. It occurs when the heart relaxes in between heart beats.

digitalis: Drug used for some cardiac arrhythmias and heart failure.

dipyridamole: The drug injected intravenously during a dipyridamole nuclear stress test. While the patient rests, dipyridamole causes a three-to fourfold increase in coronary blood flow (more than exercise does), and allows identification of coronary artery disease with greater accuracy.

diuretic: A drug that stimulates urine production. It is used in the treatment of hypertension, heart failure, or edema.

dyspnea: A shortness of breath.

echocardiography: A method of studying the heart's structure and function by analyzing sound waves bounced off the heart and recorded by an electronic sensor placed on the thorax (chest). It provides excellent information about the heart function, its chambers, heart valves and pericardium, and heart valves. *See also* cardiac ultrasound

electron beam computed tomography (EBCT): Scanning method to detect coronary artery calcifications, an important indicator of coronary artery disease, and potentially, the risk of a heart attack.

electrocardiogram (ECG): A diagnostic procedure that records the electrical activity of the heart and is useful for detection of cardiac rhythm abnormalities, acute or past myocardial infarctions, and other cardiac disorders. Also: the record of the procedure itself.

EKG: The acronym EKG is equivalent to ECG, but is formed from the German *elektrokardiogram*. *See* electrocardiogram (ECG)

edema: Abnormal accumulation of fluid in tissues due to heart failure or other causes. *See also* pulmonary edema, and leg edema

ejection fraction: The fraction (percentage) of blood ejected from the left ventricle with each cardiac beat. Normally, it is 50 percent or greater.

endocarditis: Infection of a heart valve.

endothelium: Thin layer of cells (endothelial cells) lining the inside of an artery. Maintaining the endothelium's structural integrity is crucial to avoiding arterial obstructions and clot formations.

erectile failure: Absent or diminished penile rigidity during sexual stimulation. *See* impotence

fasting cholesterol: Blood levels of cholesterol measured after fasting for twelve hours. Considered the most accurate way of determining cholesterol values.

fatty acids: Byproducts of the breakdown of various fats. When carbon molecules in fatty acids are fully occupied by hydrogen atoms, they are called saturated acids. Otherwise, they are unsaturated. *See also* hydrogenation, saturated fats, transfatty acids, and unsaturated fats

foam cells: White cells, called monocytes, that live inside the walls of arteries and migrate toward the intima sucking in large amounts of LDL cholesterol, thereby contributing to plaque formation. When the number of these cells is excessive, the atherosclerotic plaque is soft and has a greater tendency to break and form acute clots and heart attacks.

heart attack: *See* myocardial infarction

heart failure: *See* congestive heart failure

HDL: *See* high-density lipoprotein

high-density lipoprotein (HDL): The so-called "good cholesterol," which has a protective effect on the arteries. *See also* lipids, lipoproteins, low-density lipoprotein, and very-low-density lipoprotein

hydrogenation: An industrial process that adds hydrogen atoms to unsaturated fats. The purpose is to convert liquid fat into solid fat, which improves the shelf life of the product. During this process, very unhealthy transfatty acids are produced. Some margarines and commercial shortenings (used for baking cookies, pastries, cakes, doughnuts, or in cooking or frying), contain significant concentrations of transfatty acids. *See also* fats, fatty acids, saturated fats, transfatty acids, and unsaturated fats

hypotension: Abnormally low blood pressure.

impotence: See erectile failure

infarction: Permanent damage caused by a totally occluded (blocked) artery. It may occur in different organs. Examples. myocardial infarction (heart attack), cerebral infarction (stroke), spleen infarction (a clot from inside a cardiac chamber traveled down the circulation and elected to stop at the spleen station blocking one of its arteries.

inferior vena cava: The large vein that returns blood from the lower part of the body (abdomen and lower extremities) to the heart.

intima: Innermost layer of an artery. It consists of a continuous, single-cell layer of endothelial cells. *See also* foam cells

ischemia: Transient decrease in blood flow to an organ due to partial blockage of an artery. Depending upon the organ involved, different terms are used: myocardial ischemia (the heart), cerebral ischemia (the brain), renal ischemia (the kidneys), and foot ischemia (the feet), etc.

ischemic heart disease: *See* coronary heart disease

LDL: *See* low-density lipoprotein

left main artery: Vital, initial portion of the coronary arterial system.

left anterior descending artery: The largest coronary artery, which courses down the front of the heart.

left atrium: The smaller chamber of the left side of the heart that receives oxygenated blood from the lungs and passes it to the left ventricle through the mitral valve.

left circumflex coronary artery: It flexes around (circum) the left side of the heart.

left ventricle: The largest pumping chamber of the left side of the heart that ejects blood through the aorta and into circulation with each heart beat.

lipid fractions: Various fatty components of the blood lipids. *See also* lipids, and lipoproteins

lipids: Collectively, the cholesterol and its fractions, HDL, LDL, VLDL, lipoproteins, and triglycerides circulating in the blood. *See also* high-density lipoprotein, lipoproteins, low-density lipoprotein, and very-low density lipoprotein

lipoproteins: The vehicles that cholesterol and other lipid fractions use for transport in the blood. Note that triglycerides are not transported by lipoproteins. *See also* high-density lipoprotein, lipids, low-density lipoprotein, triglycerides, and very-low density lipoprotein

low–density lipoprotein: The so-called "bad cholesterol," which is coronary-unfriendly. *See also* high-density lipoprotein, lipids, lipoproteins, and very-low-density lipoprotein

lumen: Space inside a blood vessel where the blood circulates.

mitral valve: The valve that controls blood flow between the left atrium (upper chamber) and left ventricle (lower chamber).

morbidity: Complications and disabilities of a disease.

murmur: Sound detected by applying the stethoscope to the chest and that indicates the presence of a narrowed valve opening (stenosis), leaking of a valve (insufficiency or regurgitation).

myocardial infarction: Damaged area of heart muscle resulting from severe obstruction of a coronary artery. It is commonly described as a heart attack. *See also* infarction

nitric oxide (NO): Extremely important gaseous substance produced by endothelial cells; nitric oxide dilates arteries and increases blood flow.

nitroglycerin: A drug that dilate blood vessels and it is widely used to relieve anginal pains.

non–invasive procedure: Any diagnostic or treatment procedure in which no instrument enters the body.

obesity: The terms usually applies to the condition of being 30 per cent or more over one's normal body weight.

obstructive cardiomyopathy: Thick septal portion of the heart muscle that may block the exit of blood from the left ventricle, causing fainting.

pacemaker (artificial): An instrument that connects a battery-usually implanted under the clavicle or collar bone-to an electrode that stimulates the heart muscle. Its use is indicated when there is severe slowing of the heart beat; it "takes over" the cardiac rhythm when the heart itself is unable to do so. *See also* pacemaker (natural)

pacemaker (natural): The sinus node is the heart's natural pacemaker. An oval-shaped mass measuring 10-20 mm long and up to 5 mm thick, the sinus node acts like a battery. It generates an electrical impulse that is transmitted to the rest of the heart through bundles called the conducting system. This current stimulates the heart muscle, which contracts as a result. *See also* pacemaker (artificial)

penile implant: See penile prostheses

penile prostheses: A device surgically implanted inside the penis to produce rigidity.

perfusion: Blood that reaches the heart muscle.

perfusion deficit: Insufficient blood flow to certain portions of the heart muscle detected by nuclear technology.

pericarditis: Inflammation of the outer membrane surrounding the heart.

pericardium: The outer fibrous sac that sorrounds the heart.

pulmonary: Referring to the lungs.

PET *or* **PET scan.** See positron emission tomography

pharmacological stress testing: Substitute for exercise stress testing usually employed when the patient is unable to physically perform adequately.

plaque: A focalized cholesterol build-up in the inner layer of an artery.

plaque rupture: A crack in the plaque that originates the process of clot formation that blocks the artery and causes an acute myocardial infarction.

platelets: Tiny elements that "peacefully" circulate in the blood until they are "activated". This usually happens during plaque rupture. Then, they become dangerous and contribute to the formation of a clot (thrombus).

positron emission tomography (PET): Medical procedure that provides accurate, quantitative, three-dimensional pictures of blood flow in heart muscle. Also called PET scan.

progression: More severe narrowing of an artery by enlargement of an atherosclerotic plaque.

pulmonary valve: The heart valve between the right ventricle and the pulmonary artery. It controls blood flow from the heart into the lungs.

pulmonary vein: The blood vessel that carries fresh, oxygenated blood from the lungs back into the left atrium.

regression: Less severe narrowing of an artery due to atherosclerotic plaque's size reduction. In partial regression, small but very significant improvements in arterial blockages are possible when reversal therapy is applied. This treatment requires strict diet adherence and drastic lifestyle changes.

regurgitation: Term that applies to a leaking valve which is unable to close completely. As a result, some blood goes forward (which it is supposed to do), but some also goes backward (which it is not supposed to do). Consequences vary according to the valve involved and the degree of leakage. Example: If the mitral valve is insufficient, (regurgitant), blood will flow back from the left ventricle to the left atrium. If the aortic valve is insufficient, blood will flow back from the aorta to the left ventricle. When severe enough, both of the above cause increased pressure inside the lungs and shortness of breath.

renal: Pertaining to the kidneys.

reversal therapy: Method used to reduce the size of atherosclerotic plaques, diminishing the severity of arterial blockages and increasing blood flow. It combines strict dietary guidelines, medications, stress control, programmed physical exercises, etc. *See also* regression

right atrium: Small antechamber of the right side of the heart. It receives poorly oxygenated blood from the superior and inferior vena cavae and sends it to the right ventricle through the tricuspid valve.

right coronary artery: It courses around the right side of the heart to its back, or posterior surface.

right ventricle: Receives poorly oxygenated blood from the right atrium and sends it to the lungs for proper oxygenation.

risk factors: Factors that increase the risk of cardiovascular disease, including smoking, high blood pressure, and diabetes, among others.

saturated fats: Fatty acids whose carbon molecules are fully occupied by hydrogen atoms. Otherwise, they are called unsaturated. *See also* fats, fatty acids, hydrogenation, transfatty acids, and unsaturated fats

septum: The muscular tissue that divides a chamber on the left side of the heart from the chamber on the right. The muscular wall that separates both atrial chambers is called interatrial septum. The muscular wall that separates both ventricles is called interventricular septum.

sick sinus node syndrome: Failure of the sinus node to generate a normal heart beat and regulate the cardiac rhythm.

silent ischemia: Episodes of myocardial ischemia that are not accompanied by chest pain.

sinus node: *See* pacemaker (natural)

sphygmomanometer: An instrument used to measure blood pressure.

stenosis: Localized or segmental abnormal narrowing of an artery. The term also applies to diseased valves with small openings (for example, aortic stenosis, mitral stenosis). Aging and rheumatic heart disease are among the causes of valvular stenosis.

stethoscope: An instrument for listening to sounds within the body (sounds originated from the lungs, heart, and various arteries).

stent: A device made of expandable, metal mesh that is placed at the site of a narrowing artery. It is placed by using a balloon at the tip of a catheter. The stent is then expanded and kept in place to keep the artery open.

sternum: The breast bone.

stress test: Method to detect deficient blood supply to the cardiac muscle. It can be done by exercising the patient under electrocardiographic monitoring, using echocardiogram to detect ventricular wall motion abnormalities, or nuclear material injections for identification of myocardial regions that are not well perfused (not receiving the appropriate blood supply).

stroke: *See* cerebrovascular accident

superior vena cava: The large vein that returns blood from the head and upper part of the body to the heart.

supraventricular tachycardia: It is a rapid cardiac rhythm that originates above the ventricles.

syncope: A temporary loss of consciousness caused by a sudden loss of blood supply to the brain. It may result from arrhythmias, aortic stenosis, obstructive cardiomyopathy or sudden dilatation of arteries throughout the body, (due to fear, acute strong emotional reaction) among other causes.

systole: Each cardiac contraction. *See also* diastole

systolic blood pressure: The highest blood pressure measured in the arteries. It occurs when the heart contracts with each heartbeat.

tachycardia: Accelerated beating of the heart.

tachypnea: Rapid breathing.

thrombosis: A clot that forms inside an artery (arterial thrombosis) or a vein (venous thrombosis).

transesophageal echocardiography (TEE): This test is echocardiography using a tube-like device inserted in the mouth and passed down the esophagus (food pipe). In some cases, and for various reasons, it provides more accurate information than the standard echocardiography. *See also* echocardiography

transplantation: *See* cardiac transplantation

transfatty acids: Fatty acids produced during the hydrogenation process of vegetable oils, and are usually solid or semisolid at room temperature. *See also* fats, fatty acids, hydrogenation, saturated fats, and unsaturated fats

tricuspid valve: The valve that controls blood flow between the right atrium (upper chamber) and right ventricle (lower chamber).

triglycerides: A group of blood lipids that is associated with vascular disease when levels are significantly elevated. *See also* lipoproteins

thrombus: A blood clot.

thrombolysis: The breaking up of a blood clot.

thrombosis: A blood clot that forms inside the blood vessel or cavity of the heart.

thrombolytic therapy: Treatment with a drug that dissolves blood clots.

transient ischemic attack (TIA): A temporary, stroke-like event, that usually lasts from several minutes to a few hours and it is caused by a temporary blocked artery that supplies blood to the brain.

ultrasound: High-frequency sound vibrations, not audible to the human ear, used in medical diagnosis.

unsaturated fats: Fatty acids whose molecules are not fully occupied by hydrogen atoms.ions. *See also* fats, fatty acids, hydrogenation, transfatty acids, and unsaturated fats

valvular insufficiency: *See* regurgitation

varicose vein: Any vein that is abnormally dilated.

vascular: Pertaining to the blood vessels.

vein: Any blood vessel of the vascular system that carries blood from various parts of the body back to the heart. This blood has lower oxygen content than arterial blood.

vasoconstriction: Narrowing of an artery or multiple arteries throughout the arterial system, which restricts blood flow. When the constriction is limited to a small segment of an artery it is called a spasm. See also arterial spasm and vasodilation

vasodilation: Dilation of an artery, which increases blood flow. See also arterial spasm and vasoconstriction

vacuum erection device (VED): Mechanical way of producing an erection. The penis is introduced in a transparent plastic chamber of appropriate size, a little pump creates a vacuum and penis engorgement results.

valvuloplasty: Repair or reshaping of a heart valve through surgery or catheterization techniques.

ventricular fibrillation (VF): A very rapid, chaotic, ineffective cardiac rhythm.

ventricular tachycardia (VT): A fast heart beat that originates in the ventricle.

very-low-density lipoprotein (VLDL): A type of lipid that increases the risk of coronary and vascular disease. *See also* high-density lipoprotein, lipids, lipoproteins, and low-density lipoprotein

VLDL: *See* very-low-density lipoprotein

Wolff-Parkinson-White syndrome: A condition in which an abnormal electrical pathway connects the atria and the ventricles, at times causing arrhythmias.

Index

About the Author

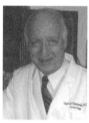

Eduardo Chapunoff, M.D. is a Diplomate of the American Board of Internal Medicine and the American Board of Cardiovascular Disease, a Fellow of the American College of Physicians and the American College of Cardiology, and a Clinical Associate Professor of Medicine at the University of Miami School of Medicine.

He has been included in the biographical records of Marquis Who's Who Publication Board, Personalities of America, Community Leaders of America (American Biographical Institute), and the International Who's Who of Intellectuals (International Biographical Centre, Cambridge, England). He was named International Man of the Year 1991-1992 (International Biographical Centre, Cambridge, England).

He is the author of *Sex and the Cardiac Patient* (1991), and its Spanish version, *El Sexo y el Paciente Cardiaco* (1992), which was also published in Argentina by Editorial Lidiun (1993). El Ateneo, one of the most prestigious publishing houses of South America, was the book's exclusive distributor. His latest book, *Morbid Obesity and the Struggle for Survival*, was published in July 2007.

Dr. Chapunoff is currently engaged in private cardiology practice with the Greater Fort Lauderdale Heart Group, Pompano Beach and Fort Lauderdale, Florida. His extra-curricular activities include violin playing and oil painting. His work has been exhibited at art galleries a number of times.

Visit his website at www.dreduardochapunoff.com